Human Immunogenetics

Principles and Clinical Applications

Human Immunogenetics
Principles and Clinical Applications

J. E. Bernal
Faculty of Medicine
Pontificia Universidad Javeriana
Bogota, Colombia

Translated from the Spanish by
Professor Derek Roberts

Department of Human Genetics
The University of Newcastle upon Tyne, England

Taylor & Francis
London and Philadelphia
1986

UK   Taylor & Francis Ltd, 4 John St, London WC1N 2ET

USA   Taylor & Francis Inc., 242 Cherry St, Philadelphia, PA 19106-1906

Orginally published in Spanish as *Genetica Immunologica* by Editorial Norma, Bogotá, Colombia. © 1982.

Revised English edition copyright © Taylor & Francis Ltd 1986.

British Library Cataloguing in Publication Data

Bernal, J. E
    Human immunogenetics: principles and
    clinical applications.
    1. Immunogenetics
    I. Title   II. Genetica immunologica.
    English
    616.07′9   QR184

    ISBN 0-85066-334-2 (pbk)
    ISBN 0-85066-355-5 (hbk)

Library of Congress Cataloging in Publication Data

Bernal, J. E (Jaime E.)
    Human immunogenetics.

    Translation of: Genetica immunologica.
    Includes bibliographies and index.
    1. Immunologic diseases—Genetic aspects.
2. Immunogenetics. I. Title. [DNLM: 1. Immunogenetics.
QW 541 B517g]
RC582.B4613   1986   616.97   86-5677
ISBN 0-85066-334-2 (pbk)
ISBN 0-85066-355-5 (hbk)

*Typeset by Mathematical Composition Setters Ltd, Salisbury, UK
Printed in Great Britain by Taylor & Francis (Printers) Ltd,
Basingstoke, Hants.*

Preface

The explosion of knowledge about the genetic mechanisms that control the human immune system has resulted in a wider application of genetic principles in clinical practice as well as in the need for those in the basic human sciences to become aquainted with immunological concepts.

Since the subject is developing at a high speed, it seemed convenient to compile some of these concepts in a readable textbook. Unavoidably, the choice of topics reflects my own interests, but I hope that those selected will be good examples of the impact of this area of biomedical research. This book has no other pretension.

I am most grateful to the many people that have contributed towards the completion of this work. My original research mentioned here has been supported by grants from Colciencias, ICFES and the Banco de la Republica in Colombia, and Colciencias also helped me in my frequent trips to the UK. I also thank the British Council for their constant interest and support throughout the years.

From my period of work in Newcastle I am greatly indebted to Professor D. F. Roberts; the years I spent there with my family are indelibly fixed in our minds, and Professor Roberts' unique ability to combine gentle manners, a sense of humour, hard work and an encyclopaedic knowledge, left a permanent imprint on me. I also thank Mrs T. Havelock for typing the manuscript and Mrs I. E. de Escallón for kindly reviewing it and making valuable comments,

Finally, my heartful thanks are to my wife, María Mercedes, our children Ana María and Alejandro, and my parents Eduardo and Consuelo for making it all worthwhile.

J. E. Bernal
Bogota
February 1986

Contents

PART I

PRINCIPLES

Chapter 1. History of immunogenetics

Of the many differences among individuals, not the least fascinating are the variations in their responses to infection. Why in the great epidemics of the past did some individuals succumb and others survive? Why today can some withstand a prophylactic inoculation without obvious ill effect, others not? Why can the life of a man be saved by a blood transfusion or a transplant from one particular individual and not from another? Considering differences between individuals has occupied thinkers since the earliest times. Opposing theories dominated philosophy, and played an important role in the development of concepts not only in biology but also in politics and religion. The concept that the individual is born as a *tabula rasa*, upon which the environment will work to determine his future, was introduced by Locke and influenced Thomas Jefferson in his conception of North American democracy. The opposite concept, that individual diversity is due entirely to genetic differences, was introduced by Plato, and taken to extremes by Calvin. Yet both are inadequate.

Present-day knowledge of the mechanism of inheritance, which is still far from complete, is the result of three centuries of research — a gradually accelerating development. The fact that biological inheritance is transmitted by germ cells was discovered only some 300 years ago. The microscope had to be invented before the existence of such cells could be confirmed. The spermatozoa were first seen by Van Leeuwenhoek in 1677. Amusingly, when Leeuwenhoek sent the results of his research to the Royal Society of London, he asked that they should not be published should they be found immoral or obscene, but stated that the material had been obtained by methods that he considered neither sinful nor contrary to good manners. The ovum was first seen in 1827 by von Baer. Meanwhile, Spallanzani's brilliant experiments had helped to elucidate the role of the spermatozoa in fertilization. He filtered dogs' semen and showed that the filtrate could not produce pregnancy. He was also the initiator of artificial insemination. Unfortunately the clarity of his experiments was not matched by equal clarity of conclusions, for from his data he deduced that the spermatozoa were essential to allow seminal fluid to induce development of the embryo.

3

This therefore was the pedigree of genetics, the conjunction of cytology with the research into inheritance initiated by Mendel. The former described cell division, chromosomes were identified, and those in the sex cells were suggested, at the end of the nineteenth century, to be the transmitters of inheritance. Mendel's writings in 1865 formulated the laws of inheritance based on his plant-hybridization studies. He showed that what is inherited is transmitted as a set of characters that in the process of formation of the germinal cells segregate and then recombine on fertilization. After Mendel's findings became accepted, inheritance was no longer considered as a blending of parental contributions, but as a mosaic of the individual factors transmitted by each. The union of the two lines of research derived from the work, at the beginning of this century, of Sutton and Boveri, who independently observed that the behaviour of the genes postulated by Mendel was similar to that of chromosomes, led to the hypothesis that genes were carried by the chromosomes.

Immunology, on the other hand, developed rapidly, arising from work on infectious diseases and bacteriology at the end of last century. The idea of a vaccine was introduced by Jenner, but this had to await Pasteur's experiments for its scientific explanation. The theory of cellular immunity developed first, thanks to the findings of Metchnikoff at the end of the nineteenth century. His followers, and those of Robert Koch, described humoral immunity mechanisms a few years later. At the beginning of this century Bordet described what we now know as the complement system, and almost at the same time Ehrlich's theory of the sidechain was introduced to explain the appearance of circulating antibodies.

It was about this time that immunology and genetics first met, when Landsteiner described the ABO blood groups. Knowing that a reaction occurred when blood from different species was mixed, Landsteiner looked for similar reactions between individuals of the same species, and found that some combinations were followed by red blood cell agglutination. In 1901 he announced the theory of agglutinogens and agglutinins. Ottenberg and Epstein (1908) were the first to suggest a hereditary basis to the blood groups, although their data were not sufficiently complete to be convincing. However, von Dungern and Hirschfeld (1910) succeeded in confirming this hypothesis. Knowledge of the blood groups has since come a long way, and today serology is a vast field with many practical applications in genetics and immunology.

Once the inheritance of the blood groups was defined in Mendelian terms, and with the identity of genetic constitution of monozygous twins already established, it was only one step further to discover that other tissue differences might be inherited as well. This step was taken by Gibson and Medawar when in 1943 they reported their observations on the behaviour of skin grafts in a child, thus opening the door to research into tissue rejection and the diversity of cellular and tissue antigens, especially those governing histocompatibility.

In the past few years, many crucial discoveries have placed the major histocompatibility complex at a much higher level of biological importance than was initially thought. The first important advance was the characterization of congenic strains of mice that differed only in parts of their system of histocompatibility antigens (H-2). This work was largely due to Gores and Snell, and was the basis for the study of the genetic control of immune responses to well-defined antigens, many of which have since been shown to be associated with the major histocompatibility complex (MHC). This has been principally the contribution of Benacerraf. The second advance came with the initial studies of the cells involved in the immune system, followed by the study of T and B lymphocytes, their interaction, and the role of the macrophage. Possibly the third major area of advance was the chromosomal assignment of the genes involved in the immune response, following an enormous amount of work dedicated to the linkage between these and other genes, and associations between these genes and particular diseases. The characterization of the products of these genes was a major contribution of Dausset. Snell, Benacerraf and Dausset shared the Nobel Prize in 1980 for their pioneering work in this field.

The first indication that the complement system was controlled by the MHC was in the mouse. In 1973 it was demonstrated that the substance Ss, coded by the S region of the H-2, was a component of murine complement. This led to intensive work on the genetics of complement, and a genetic element has been established in the control of the majority of its components studied so far.

Other important interactions between immunology and genetics were initiated by the work of Waller, who reported the presence of a factor in the serum of arthritic patients, capable of agglutinating goat red cells covered with low doses of anti-erythrocyte antibodies. In 1956 Grubb noticed that the same type of serum was capable of agglutinating Rh-positive red cells coated with incomplete anti-Rh antibodies. The factor responsible for this activity was named Gm(a). Other Gm factors were subsequently discovered, known today as allotypic determinants associated with the immunoglobulin chains, and these are genetically controlled and have been widely applied in studies of population genetics.

Finally, other important concepts have emerged out of the fusion of genetics and immunology. The theory of tolerance proposed by Medawar and Burnet, the understanding of chimerism, the first description of agammaglobulinaemia followed by the discovery of other immune deficiency diseases, are just a few examples of fields that are today objects of intense research activity.

As a result, immunogenetics in man has emerged as a subdiscipline in its own right. It has given understanding of the aetiology of a whole group of formerly little-understood diseases and the mechanisms contributing to them — the auto-immune disorders. It has allowed the development of the critical life-saving procedures of transplantation of tissues and organs. It has produced the tools, techniques and models to be validated by animal experiment, which have made such an impact on modern medicine.

6   *Human immunogenetics*

Bibliography

Demant, P., Capkova, J. and Hinzova, E., 'The role of the histocompatibility-2-linked Ss-Slp region in the control of mouse complement. *Proc. Natl Acad. Sci. USA,* **70**: 863 (1973).

Dobzansky, T., *Evolution, Genetics and Man.* John Wiley, New York (1955).

Dunn, L. C., *A Short History of Genetics.* McGraw-Hill, New York (1965).

Foster, W. D., *History of Medical Bacteriology and Immunology.* Heinemann, London (1970).

Gibson, T. and Medawar, P. B., Fate of skin homografts in man. *J. Anat.*, **77**: 299 (1943).

Grubb, R. Agglutination of erythrocytes coated with 'incomplete' anti-Rh by certain rheumatoid arthritic sera and some other sera: the existance of human serum groups. *Acta Pathol. Microbiol. Scand.*, **39**: 195 (1956).

Landsteiner, K., *The Specificity of Serological Reactions.* Thomas, Illinois (1936).

McKusick, V. A., The growth and development of human genetics as a clinical discipline. *Am. J. Hum. Genet.*, **27**: 261–273 (1975)

Ottenberg, R. and Epstein, A. A., A method for hemolysis and agglutination tests. *Arch. Intern. Med.*, iii: 286 (1908).

Scriver, C. R., Genetics and Medicine: an evolving relationship. *Science*, **200**: 946 (1978).

Stern, C. and Sherwood, E. R. (eds), *The Origin of Genetics. A Mendel Source Book.* W. H. Freeman, San Francisco (1966).

von Dungern, E. and Hirschfeld, L., Ueber eine Method, das Blut verschiedener Menschen serologisch zu unterscheiden. *Munch. Med. Wochenschr.*, vii: 741 (1910).

Chapter 2. A general view of the immune system

In this chapter an attempt is made to summarize in a few pages the most important features of how the immune system functions. Since the explanation of many of these topics requires some knowledge of the rudiments of immunogenetics, cross reference is made to those chapters that contain more details on each topic. To avoid interruptions of sequence, definitions of new terms are given in the Glossary, pp. 205–211.

The immune system is generally thought of as consisting of two components: one influenced by the thymus and responsible for cellular immunity, and the other responsible for humoral immunity, which is under the influence of the bursa of Fabricius in birds and of organs of equivalent function in mammals. Although there is good evidence of this basic dual nature in man, the true situation is more complex, and interaction between the two components is important.

There are two steps in the development and expression of the immune response. First, a set of immunocompetent cells is generated under the influence of the primary lymphoid organs, independent of the presence or absence of any antigenic stimulation. Thereafter these differentiated cells migrate to the secondary lymphoid organs where, if they have come into contact with an antigen, they proliferate and initiate a series of events that lead to the elimination of the antigenic material. A simplified scheme of this immune response can be seen in Figure 2.1.

2.1. Differentiation of T and B lymphocytes

The lymphoid system in man is characterized by the presence of two major populations of immunocompetent lymphocytes, morphologically indistinguishable but with different surface components and antigenic markers. Generally speaking these are responsible for the two main types of immune response. One, mediated by the T lymphocytes, is involved in allotransplant rejection, graft-versus-host disease, contact sensitivity, and reaction to certain viral, fungal and

7

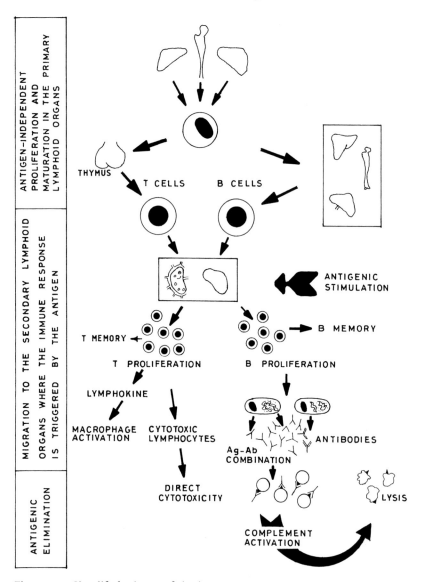

Figure 2.1. Simplified scheme of the immune response.

protozoal infections. The other type involving the B lymphocytes is more important in immediate hypersensitivity reactions, some bacterial and viral infections
and immune complex diseases. These cells interact however, and T cells mediate
a number of B-cell functions.

These two types of cell mature by a process of cellular differentiation that starts
in the yolk sac of the embryo. This yolk sac is the place where the primordial cells

of the haematopoietic system proliferate and then differentiate into a variety of blood cells, including lymphocytes. When maturation in the yolk sac ceases, the foetal liver, spleen and bone marrow become the major sites of prenatal synthesis; later, in the postnatal period, the bone marrow becomes the main centre of this activity.

From these primary lymphoid organs, the primitive cells of the immune system migrate to other sites, where differentiation of T and B lymphocytes occurs. In man, the serious impairment of T-cell functions in congenital thymic aplasia shows the important role of this organ in promoting the development and maturation of T cells. However, cells with T markers have been observed in athymic (nu/nu) mice suggesting, as some other studies seem to confirm, that a very small proportion of T lymphocytes may differentiate in the absence of the thymus. It seems that there are two types of T cell in the developing thymus: one, which predominates in the cortex, involves prothymocytes and thymocytes containing a DNA polymerase called terminal deoxynucleotidyl transferase (TdT + cells), and another without this enzyme which predominates in the thymic medulla (TdT -). It is not clear whether these two types of cell give rise to different subpopulations of T lymphocytes.

There are three hypothetical stages of intrathymic differentiation of T lymphocytes. First the large thymic blasts, TdT + , which do not express markers of mature lymphocytes. Then the cortical thymocyte, still TdT + but weaker, expressing more of the adult-type determinants. Finally the medullary mature thymocyte, TdT - , which receives some influence from a HLA-DR-positive macrophage-like cell (interdigitating cell) in its final maturation into a T cell.

There are various other mechanisms that seem to play a role in the development of T lymphocytes. There is a substance in the thymus of the mouse (thymosin) that can cause surface antigens to appear, thus promoting the formation of rosettes of immature lymphoid cells. Other humoral factors probably involved include thymin (or thymopoietin), the humoral factor of the thymus (the thymic factor) and the thymus-replacement factor. Some hormonal systems are also important in the differentiation of not only T but also B lymphocytes. For example, hypocalcaemia results in abnormal behaviour of T cells, and the somatotrophic hormone intensifies the participation of T cells in the graft-versus-host reactions. From calf serum two substances capable of inducing lymphopoiesis have been isolated, and named lympho-stimulating hormones.

The maturation of the other cellular arm of the immune system, the B cell, is equally complex. The bone-marrow lymphocytes are divided into two different populations: a major proportion is short-lived and of local origin, while a minor group is long-lived and comes from the circulatory stream. Among those of local origin in the bone marrow are those believed to be the B-cell precursors. These precursors do not have immunoglobulin on their surface (sIg⁻), whose presence is the major characteristic of B cells. Nevertheless, the progeny of these pre-B cells develop surface immunoglobulin a few days after migrating to the spleen. However, the pre-B cells can be identified by the presence of cytoplasmic immunoglobulin (IgM), and these cells have been observed in the foetal mouse liver as early as the twelfth day of gestation and in the human embryo at around the seventh week of gestation. This process of maturation from negative cytoplasmic IgM (cIg$^-$) to sIg$^+$ is controlled by mechanisms that are not well known. The lymphocyte-activating factor (interleukin-1), accessory T cells, and the T-cell growth factor (interleukin-2) seem to play a role in inducing this process. Part of the differentiation of the B lymphocytes is mirrored by the sequential expression of the immunoglobulin genes (see p. 27).

2.2. *Behaviour of the immunocompetent cells*

Surface receptors

The immune response is potentially a destructive weapon and hence needs to be selective. One can think of this selectivity in terms of specific antibodies, with a receptor site on their surface capable of combining with only a limited number of antigenic determinants. In B cells the surface receptors include therefore the expression on their membrane of the gene that codes for the variable region of the immunoglobulin. However, this concept is not as simple as it first appears (see p. 27).

There are mainly two immunoglobulins (isotypes), IgD and IgM, present on the membrane of B lymphocytes. The many IgD and IgM molecules present on the surface of a single lymphocyte have identical variable regions (V) in both the heavy (H) and the light (L) chains (see p. 24). When such a cell finds its 'perfect' antigen, it proliferates, differentiates into a plasma cell and produces an immunoglobulin with the same antigenic specificity as that in its membrane. The basic mechanism underlying this combination of identical V regions in different immunoglobulin classes is a switch that operates during differentiation of the B cell (see Chapter 3).

Similarly, there exist surface receptors on T cells for the recognition of specific antigens and cell-to-cell interactions. In view of the antigenic specificity of T and B cells and the property of immunoglobulins of recognizing antigens, it appeared logical to conclude that the immunoglobulins were among the antigenic receptors of both types of lymphocyte. In fact, anti-light-chain antibodies have been shown to inhibit T-cell reactions, which led for some time to the belief that T lymphocytes bear complete immunoglobulin molecules on their surface. Recent studies have shown, however, by means of serological and molecular analysis, that the T-cell antigen receptor comprises two glycosylated, disulphide-linked polypeptide chains (α and β), both spanning the cell membrane. Although these proteins are not immunoglobulins, the genes coding the T-cell receptor show the same structure and behaviour as immunoglobulin genes, indicating some evolutionary relationship (see Chapter 5).

The T and B cells also have other series of surface receptors and antigens. The

Table 2.1.. T-cell subpopulations in mouse and man.

	Mouse	Man
Helper T cells	Lyt-1^+, 2^-, 3^-	$T3^+$, $T4^+$, $T8^-$
Cytotoxic T cells	Lyt-$1^{+/-}$, 2^+, 3^+	$T4^-$, $T8^+$
Suppressor T cells	Lyt-1^-, 2^+, 3^+	$T4^-$, $T8^+$

majority of B lymphocytes have a receptor for antigen–antibody complexes and for immunoglobulins, known as the Fc receptor. There are also receptors for several of the complement components (C3b, C3d) on some of the B cells.

The first indication that human T lymphocytes have a variety of functions came from the finding that T cells forming rosettes with IgM-coated ox red blood cells had stimulator effects on the B-cell synthesis of immunoglobulins, while T cells forming rosettes with IgG-coated cells had a suppressive effect. The introduction of murine monoclonal antibodies has given a better tool for identifying human T lymphocytes. General T lymphocytes react with monoclonal antibody against the T3 determinant, helper lymphocytes react with T4 antibodies but fail to do so with T8, and suppressor T cells do the converse ($T4^-$, $T8^+$). There is therefore a correspondence between the human T subpopulations detected by the monoclonal antibodies, and the murine T cells detected by their expression of Lyt antigens as observed in Table 2.1.

The development of other monoclonal antibodies has shown that populations of the T lymphocytes in this classification are still functionally heterogeneous. Further changes are therefore to be expected on this point.

Curious data are also coming from similar studies on the B lymphocyte. Here again, a whole variety of antigens has been detected in the murine model, but so far no clear sub-population has been identified. The Lyb-2 antigen for instance is solely confined to B lymphocytes and seems to operate in the triggering of B cells by T-dependent antigens. This antigen and another, the PC.1, seem to be mutally exclusive proteins expressed in sequence on the B-cell membrane. Another system of potential interest is the 'lymph node antigen 1' (Lna-1), as it is present only on those T and B lymphocytes that are found in the lymph nodes. It is possible, according to some data, that this antigen is confined to the lympho-cytes in the spleen and its study may therefore give some clues to the immu-nological role of this organ.

Genetic control and intracellular events

Any individual is likely to be exposed to a great variety of antigenic substances, against which he or she will need to produce a corresponding great variety of specific immune proteins (immunoglobulins and surface receptors). Such molecular diversity within the individual is unique, and hence the genetic control of these specialized types of proteins differs from any other enzyme or protein in the organism. As will be described in detail later (Chapter 3), each molecule of immunoglobulin is made up of two heavy (H) and two light (L) chains. A region of about 110 amino acids from the amino terminal of both H and L chains is particularly important because it contributes to the heterogeneity of the antibody population through variations in its amino acid. This is known as the variable or V region. In the tertiary structure of the immunoglobulins, these V regions form the domain of the immunoglobulin molecule that has the specific function of binding the antigen. The rest of the polypeptide, with the exception of the allotypic differences, is relatively constant, and is known therefore as the constant or C region.

The mechanisms of synthesis and secretion of immunoglobulins have been studied in detail. The H and L chains are produced separately in the polyribosomes of the endoplasmic reticulum. Once liberated, H–H dimers are formed, followed by an intermediate, H$_2$L, structure and finally the complete immunoglobulin molecule takes shape. IgA and IgM are polymers, and polymerization seems to occur just after secretion (although the IgM of non-stimulated B cells is not in polymeric form). This polymerization is associated with the addition of another polypeptide, the J chain. It seems for instance that there is some further assembly after the immunoglobulin (particularly for IgA) has been secreted by the B cell, in which there is a combination with the secretor component, an epithelial product. This component may play a part in the movement of IgA towards the secretory surfaces, but may also confer some resistance on the immunoglobulin, making it less susceptible to proteolytic digestion.

Cell interactions

The whole process of B-cell maturation that leads to the production of an adequate antibody is regulated both positively and negatively by a network of interacting agents. Many antigens require the co-operation of helper T cells for the B cell to produce a maximal immune response. On the other hand, suppressor T cells may also inhibit the production of immunoglobulins (Figure 2.2).

In a general sense the cell interactions that take part in the immune response either require a cell-to-cell contact or are mediated by soluble factors released by one of the cells involved. The T–B co-operation seems to fall within the former group, not requiring, therefore, the liberation of specific factors. This interaction also involves T helper cells specific for the antigen as well as the antigenic determinant (idiotype) of the B cells.

On the other hand, the co-operation between T lymphocytes has been studied through cytolytic effector lymphocytes that can be analysed directly by a cytotoxicity assay. As in T–B lymphocyte collaboration, the development of cytotoxic responses requires interactions between subsets of different T-cell types. Various steps are known to take place. First, the antigen reacts with the antigen-specific T-cell receptor, which is in itself functionally dual, since it recognizes the foreign

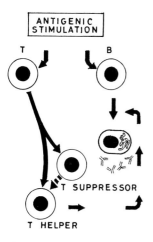

Figure 2.2. Mechanisms of cell co-operation.

antigen but only in the context of the self-antigens (H-2 or HLA-A, B, C). This reaction with the antigen activates the T lymphocyte expressing another receptor with specificity for the interleukin (Il-2), which is a growth hormone-like molecule released by helper T lymphocytes. For the helper T lymphocyte to produce the Il-2, a similar reaction with antigen has to take place, this time the antigen being presented by the macrophage which releases the other interleukin (Il-1). Yet for the T cell to become a full cytotoxic cell a third lymphokine has to be released (cytotoxic-T-lymphocyte differentiation factor) whose molecular nature and mode of action have not yet been defined. New terminology has been introduced recently for the antigens on the surface of the T cell, after studies using monoclonal antibodies. These molecules have been grouped in 'clusters of differentiation' as in Table 2.2.

A point to stress here is the necessity for the immune system to recognize

Table 2.2. Clusters of differentiation (CD) according to the Second Workshop on the Human Leukocyte Differentiation Antigens.

CD	Synonym
CD1	T6, Leu 6
CD2	T11, LFA-2, SRBC receptor
CD3	T3, Leu 4
CD4	T4, Leu 3
CD5	T1, Leu 1
CD6	T12
CD8	T8, Leu 2
CD25	Tac, Il-2 receptor

foreign antigens only in the context of its own antigens. The mechanism of this restriction of the immune response will be developed in Chapter 5.

Finally, cellular co-operation in the immune response is not only quantitatively but also qualitatively important. It has been observed for instance that T-cell-dependent B-cell activation induces an IgG response dominated by IgG1-producing cells, while the T-cell-independent B-cell activation results in an IgG3 predominant response.

2.3. Amplification system

The combination of the antigen with an appropriate antibody is followed by a series of events that lead to the elimination of the foreign material. The T cell usually produces a series of mediators whose activities increase or regulate the immune response. On the other hand, the combination of antigen and antibody induces conformational changes that allow it to activate the complement system, resulting in a series of events tending to eliminate the invading cells or bacteria.

The complement system itself poses interesting problems from both the immunological and the genetic points of view. The various components of this system circulate normally as functionally inactive molecules in pro-enzyme form, but can be activated in a cascade fashion, each component being activated in sequence under appropriate conditions. The most important of the several components is the activated complex of the last five components that together act as a unit to attack the cellular membrane, so bringing about bacteriolysis or immune haemolysis. There are two independent routes for the activation and formation of this complex of terminal components (Figure 2.3). In the classical pathway, the components involved are C1, C4, C2 and C3. The component C1 is an assemblage of three subunits C1q, C1r and C1s in a molecular ratio of 1 : 2 : 4. These subunits are joined together by non-covalent bridges through calcium ions. The recognition unit of the C1 component is the molecule of C1q that binds part of the non-variable portion of the antibody, the Fc region (see p. 19), after the conformational changes induced in it by its combination with the antigen. The activation of this C1 component is a property of IgM and IgG, the former being a thousand times more potent than the latter since only one molecule of IgM is necessary for the combination with C1, while two adjacent molecules of IgG are necessary for the same union.

Component C4 is the natural substrate for the C1s enzyme. By hydrolytic proteolysis, the C4 molecule is broken down into two fragments: a small C4a and a large activated C4b. The latter hydrolyses C2, producing C2b and C2a. After the combination of C2a with C4b, an active enzyme is formed, C4b 2a. Its substrate is C3, which is broken into two fragments: a larger one of molecular weight 175 000 capable of binding cell-surface receptors, and the smaller C3a which is a potent anaphylatoxin and chemotactic factor.

This activation of C3 can also be induced by another mechanism — the alter-

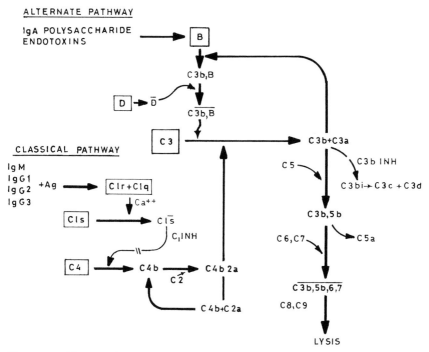

Figure 2.3. The complement system.

nate or properdin pathway discovered by Pillemer *et al.* in 1954. In this pathway the presence of antibody is not essential, and hence it is useful in the initial phases of infection when no specific antibodies are available. The basic requirement of the alternate pathway is an activated C3 molecule. There are various immunological factors that can activate C3 and hence initiate the alternate pathway. Among them are the immunoglobulins A, E and G, enzymes like trypsin, lipopolysaccharides, bacterial polysaccharides, and the cobra venom factor. Two further components of this pathway are factor B (C3 pro-activator) and factor D. The interaction of C3b, factor B and factor D forms a complex on the cell surface; D activates B, breaking it down into two parts, one of which (Bb activated) acts upon C3 to produce activated C3b; hence a feedback mechanism occurs. The activation of C5 can then be induced by either pathway, and is the last enzymatic reaction in the activation sequence of the complement system. The remaining components, C6, C7, C8 and C9, combine to form a multimolecular complex that brings about cellular lysis.

Natural control of complement activation

Complement activation is a complex process. It produces a shower of activated fragments and hence control mechanisms are needed to prevent adverse effects.

This control comes by two mechanisms: spontaneous decay of the fragments and activation of inhibitors. Included in the latter mechanisms are the inhibitor of C1 (C1 esterase inhibitor) that inhibits the action of C1s by stoichiometric combination with it, and the C3b inactivator (KAF) that stops the action of C3b by breaking it into two smaller fragments. Other inactivators have been described, but await further characterization.

2.4. Summary

This very simplified scheme of the immune response shows the complex network of interacting agents necessary for dealing correctly with a foreign antigen. It also shows that most of the antigen-independent, as well as dependent, events that take place are well controlled by genetic mechanisms, from the timed expression of surface antigens by a given set of cells to its recognition, in interplay with a foreign antigen, by another distinct cellular population. The following chapters deal with the genetic mechanisms that operate at all these levels.

Bibliography

Adinolfi, M., Haddad, S. A. and Seller, M. J., X Chromosome complement and serum levels of IgM in man and mouse. *J. Immunogenet.*, **5**: 149 (1978).

Ballieux, R. E. and Heiznen, C. J., Immunoregulatory T cell subpopulations in man: dissection by monoclonal antibodies and Fc-receptors. *Immunological Rev.*, **74**: 5 (1983).

Bernal, J. E. and Wagstaff, T. I., Cord serum AFP and the immunological status of the mother. A lack of correlation. *Biol. Neonate*, **37**: 297 (1980).

Bottomly, K., Jones, B., Kaye, J. and Jones III, F., Subpopulations of B cells distinguished by cell surface expression of Ia antigens: correlation of Ia and idiotype during activation by cloned Ia-restricted T cells. *J. Exp. Med.*, **158**: 265 (1983).

Coutinho, A. and Meo, T., Immunoglobulin gene expression by T lymphocytes. *Scand. J. Immunol.*, **18**: 79 (1983).

Freedman, M. H., Raff, M. D. and Compters, B., Induction of increased calcium uptake and its modulation by cyclic nucleotides. *Nature (Lond.)*, **255**: 378 (1975).

Gathings, W. E., Cooper, M. D., Lawton, A. R. and Alford, C. A. B cell ontogeny in humans. *Fed. Proc.*, **35**: 276 (abstract) (1976).

Goldstein, G., Isolation of bovine thymin: a polypeptide hormone of the thymus. *Nature (Lond.)*, **247**: (1974).

Kabat, E. A., *Structural Concepts in Immunology and Immunochemistry*. Holt, Rinehart and Winston, New York (1976).

Katz, D. H. and Benacerraf, B., The function and interrelationship of T-cell receptors, Ir genes and other histocompatibility gene products. *Transplant. Rev.*, **22**: 175 (1974).

Komuro, K. and Boyse, E. A., Induction of T lymphocytes from precursor cells *in vitro* by a product of the thymus. *J. Exp. Med.*, **138**: 479 (1973).

McConnell, I., Munro, A. and Waldmann, H. (eds), *The Immune System*, 2nd edition. Blackwell Scientific, Oxford (1981).

Miller, J. F. A. P., The biology of the T cell in the mouse. *Pathology.*, **14**: 395 (1982).

Osmond, D. G. and Nossal, G. J. V., Differentiation of lymphocytes in bone marrow. II. Kinetics of maturation and renewal of antiglobulin-binding cells studied by double labelling. *Cell Immunol.*, **13**: 132 (1974).

Owen, J. J. T., Cooper, M. D. and Raff, M. C., *In vitro* generation of B lymphocytes in mouse fetal liver, a mammalian 'bursa equivalent'. *Nature (Lond.)*, **249**: 361 (1974).

Pierpaoli, W., Baroni, C., Fabris, N. and Sortein, E., Hormones and immunological capacity. II. Reconstitution of antibody production in hormonally deficient mice by somatotropic hormone. *Immunology*, **16**: 217 (1969).

Pillemer, L., Blum, L., Lepow, I. H., Ross, O. A., Todd, E. W. and Wardlow, A. C., The properdin system and immunity. I. Demonstration and isolation of a new serum protein, properdin, and its role in immune phenomena. *Science*, **120**: 279 (1954).

Roelants, G. E., Loor, F., Von Boehmer, H., Haas, L., Mayor, K. S. and Ryden, A., Five types of lymphocytes characterised by double immunofluorescence in normal and nude mice. *Eur. J. Immunol.*, **5**: 127 (1975).

Rowe, D. S., Hug, K., Forni, L. and Pernis, B., Immunoglobulin D as a lymphocyte receptor. *J. Exp. Med.*, **138**: 965 (1973).

Shen, F., Yakura, H. and Tung, J. Some compartments of B cell differentiation. *Immunological Rev.*, **69**: 68 (1982).

Shimonkevitz, R., Kappler, J., Marrack, P. and Grey, H., Antigen recognition by H-2 restricted T cells: I-cell-free antigen processing. *J. Exp. Med.*, **158**: 303 (1983)

Stiehm, E. R. and Fulginiti, V. A., *Immunologic Disorders in Infants and Children*. W. B. Saunders, Philadelphia (1973).

Swain, S. L., T cell subsets and the recognition of MHC class. *Immunological Rev.*, **74**: 129 (1983).

Taussing, M. J., Mozes, E. and Isac, R., Antigen-specific thymic cell factors in the genetic control of the immune response to Poly (Tyrosil, glutamyl)-poly-D, L-alanyl-poly-lysil. *J. Exp. Med.*, **140**: 301 (1974).

Waldmann, T. A., Korsmeyer, S. J., Hieter, P. A., Ravetch, J. V., Broder, S. and Leder, P., Regulation of the humoral immune response: from immunoglobulin genes to regulatory T cell networks. *Fed. Proc.*, **42**: 2498 (1983).

Chapter 3. The structure and genetics of the immunoglobulin molecule

The immunoglobulins, varied as they are, all have one feature in common: their basic structure. Knowledge of this structure has been much advanced by the study of myelomas, in which a great number of cells are derived from a single ancestral cell to produce a single antibody, for this is similar to the production of immunoglobulins, which are also homogeneous substances. Figure 3.1 shows the basic structure of one molecule of immunoglobulin G (IgG) as proposed by Edelman and Porter, but it is used here to show properties typical of every immunoglobulin. An immunoglobulin molecule is made up of four chains: two heavy (H) and two light (L) joined by disulphide bridges. Although the molecules are in general resistant to proteolytic digestion, the enzyme papain breaks them into three fragments: two Fab fragments, capable of binding antigenic deter-

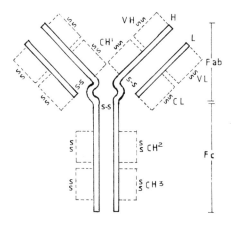

Figure 3.1. Basic structure of the immunoglobulin molecule.

minants, and one Fc fragment. The Fab and Fc fragments join in what is known as the 'hinge' region. One Fab fragment contains one L chain and approximately half of one H chain (the Fd fragment). This unit of four chains, then, is the basic structure of every immunoglobulin.

3.1. Immunoglobulin classes

The major classes of human immunoglobulins are IgG, IgA, IgM, IgD and IgE. The last two are present only in small quantities in serum. The basic difference between these five immunoglobulins is the specificity of their H chains, which are of five types (γ, α, μ, δ and ε). A molecule of IgG is made up, then, of two H chains of the γ class and two L chains; one molecule of IgD is made up of two H chains of the δ class plus two L chains. There is, however, further variation, since the light chains can be of two types: λ and $\varkappa$. While H chains are specific for each immunoglobulin, light chains are not, and hence an H chain can join any light chain of the λ or $\varkappa$ type, but not both in the same molecule. There are further differences between the immunoglobulins. IgD, IgE and IgG are found in serum as a unit of four chains, but IgA and IgM have special organization. In serum, IgM is found as a polymer of five units of four chains each, joined by disulphide bridges. IgA is not only found in serum, but is also the main immunoglobulin in secretions, and it is present in various forms. In serum it is usually present as a unit of four chains, but it can be polymerized to form larger structures of two, four or more basic units joined by disulphide bridges. In secretions, this immunoglobulin is found as a dimer, but it includes another protein, the secretory component, that is synthesized by the secretory cells binding the IgA molecule through disulphide bridges. This component seems to be necessary in the protection of the immunoglobulin against the external environment. Another polypeptide found in association with the immunoglobulins is the J chain which is invariably found in the polymeric forms of IgA and IgM. This J chain is produced by the antibody-producing cells, but its gene is located on a different chromosome from those that code for the immunoglobulin chains.

Immunoglobulin subclasses

The genetics of immunoglobulin would be simple if the variation in its structure were confined to what has so far been described. There are further factors to take into account. The evolution by gene duplication of some of the heavy chains has produced subclasses that differ in their amino acid sequences and biological properties. Four subclasses of γ chains (that of IgG) have been identified, γ_1, γ_2, γ_3 and γ_4, producing therefore four IgG subclasses: IgG1, IgG2, IgG3 and IgG4. Sequencing the amino acids of this chain has demonstrated that the subclasses are very similar, being between 70 and 90% homologous. All these subclasses are present in any individual. Similarly, two subclasses have also been identified in

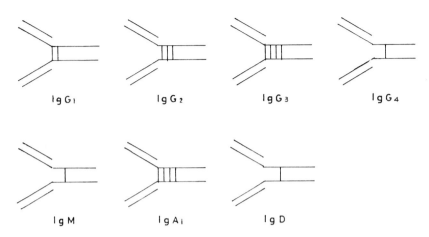

Figure 3.2. Distribution of disulphide bridges in some classes of immunoglobulins.

the α chain and perhaps the μ chain, and it seems likely that subclasses will be identified for the other heavy chains. The immunoglobulin subclasses differ not only in their amino acid sequences and chemical properties, but also in the distribution of disulphide bridges. Figure 3.2 shows the position of these bridges in some of the immunoglobulin classes and subclasses.

Of the two classes of light chains, similar variation has been observed in only one of them. The human λ chain exists in four forms, depending on the presence or absence of two antigenic determinants called Kern and Oz. These antigenic determinants are the result of a small number of amino acid substitutions. The Oz(+) chains have lysine and the Oz(−) have arginine at position 188. the Kern(+) chains have glycine while Kern(−) have serine at position 157. the resultant chains are therefore of four types: Ke^-Oz^-; Ke^+Oz^-; Ke^-Oz^+; Ke^+Oz^+. Three of these have so far been observed. There is still another variant of this light chain, named λ_{Mcg}, that has asparagine, threonine and lysine instead of alanine, serine and tyrosine at positions 111, 113 and 167, respectively.

Variable and constant regions

The final source of variation in immunological structure was shown by primary amino acid sequencing of light and heavy chains. When the first light chains were so studied, it was observed that the residues 1–108 varied frequently from protein to protein within the groups of $\varkappa$ and λ chains, while the other residues were fairly constant (from 109 to 215). These two regions of the light chains are now known respectively as the V, or variable, and C, or constant, regions.

Heavy chains are also made up of V and C regions, the variable region being of similar size to that in the light chains. Disulphide bridges play an important role in the secondary structure of these proteins. In each light chain there are two of these bridges, four in the heavy chains of type γ, α and δ, and five in the μ and ε heavy chains. These bridges give loop conformations of about 60–70 amino acid residues that are quite peculiar. Sequencing of these loops shows that in the heavy chain they are quite similar amongst themselves, with a homology that extends over the region of the disulphide bridges to cover a total of about 110 amino acids. These homologous regions are called domains. There is, however, little homology between the domains of the C and V region, while it is very marked between all domains of the C region. In the γ chain, the homologous region of the amino terminal is known as V_H and the other three homologous regions, located in the C region, are called $C\gamma_1$, $C\gamma_2$ and $C\gamma_3$. It has been suggested that each of these domains is responsible for one of the specific biological properties of the immunoglobulins. It is now established that the variable region of the immunoglobulin provides the basis of its immunological specificity.

It is necessary to add one more concept about immunoglobulin structure variation. There are three regions in the V portion of the light and heavy chains that show even more variation, known as complementary-determining regions (or hypervariable regions): CDR_1, CDR_2 and CDR_3. The rest of the variable portion of both chains consist of four regions flanking the CDRs and referred to as framework regions, FR_1, FR_2, FR_3 and FR_4. The CDR_3 of the heavy chains at the gene level is usually referred to as the D region, while the FR_4 of both light and heavy chains forms the J region. That is to say, besides the variable and constant regions, the light chain genes have a J region, three other framework regions and three complementarity-determining regions.

3.2. Biological properties of the immunoglobulins

The basic structure of the immunoglobulin molecule, the processes by which the five classes of immunoglobulins are produced, the variations in light chains, the subsequent division in subclasses of light and heavy chains, and finally the presence of the constant, variable and hypervariable regions for the high specificity of the antibodies, all affect the biological properties of these proteins.

Table 3.1. Some biological properties of the immunoglobulins.

Immunoglobulin	Heavy chain MW	Whole molecule MW	Complement fixation	Serum concentration (mg / 100 ml)
IgM	70 000	900 000	+	60–200
IgG	50 000	150 000	+	800–1600
IgA	55 000	$(160\,000)^n$	–	150–400
IgD	65 000	180 000	?	3
IgE	65 000	180 000	–	0.05

Obviously, the most important main functions of the immunoglobulins are combination with antigens, but some other functions have been ascribed to them (Table 3.1).

Immunoglobulin G

This is the immunoglobulin present in highest concentration in serum. One important function of this immunoglobulin is the protection of the newborn, since maternal IgG can cross the placenta during the last trimester of pregnancy so that the newborn usually has IgG levels equal to or even higher than those of the mother. Contrary to what was initially thought, all the IgG classes can cross the placenta, and IgG1 and IgG3 are capable of activating the complement system through the classical pathway.

The ability of IgG to reach the extra-vascular space makes it a very efficient agent in the neutralization of bacterial exotoxins. It can also promote phagocytosis by two mechanisms: one using the C3b receptor on the macrophage, and the other by direct union of the IgG to the surface of the macrophage at its receptor.

Immunoglobulin A

This is the main immunoglobulin in exocrine secretions where it is found as a dimer, while in serum it is found as a basic monomer. Aggregated IgA is capable of activating the complement system through the alternate pathway, and it can therefore induce phagocytosis and activate the macrophage. There is no evidence, however, of this immunoglobulin producing opsonification. Secretory IgA blocks bacterial adherence to mucosal surfaces, thus preventing colonization. The molecule is quite resistant to proteolysis, which is probably due to its combination with the secretory component; this is a real advantage in an environment such as the gastrointestinal tract.

Immunoglobulin M

Although its serum concentration is relatively low, IgM is often the first immunoglobulin in the response to antigenic stimulation. It is very effective in activating the complement system, particularly when combined with cell-membrane antigens.

Perhaps of more importance is its ability to promote immune adherence to phagocytic cells, an activity that is mediated by the complement system. Although it is not capable of opsonification, it can induce phagocytosis through its activation of the complement system. High levels of this immunoglobulin in the neonatal period are an indication of intrauterine infection.

Immunoglobulin D

The role of this immunoglobulin is not yet clear, and there is no evidence that it is specific for any antigen. IgD does not cross the placental barrier, neither does it activate the complement system, but on the other hand it is found on the surface of B lymphocytes during ontogeny, which suggests that it may play a role in the induction of immune tolerance.

Immunoglobulin E

This immunoglobulin mediates the majority of allergic reactions. Its serum concentration is very low (of the order of nanograms per millilitre) and almost all the protein is to be found on the surface of basophils and mast cells. On the surface of these cells, the union of the antigen to IgE molecules is enough to trigger the biochemical events leading to the liberation of histamine, SRS-A and ECF-A. These substances are responsible for the majority of the phenomena observed in the IgE-mediated immune responses.

The correlation between atopic diseases and high IgE levels is well known, but not all the allergic diseases produce a similar increase in IgE levels: the increase is pronounced in atopic eczema, but is only moderate in extrinsic asthma. Some parasitic diseases also induce high levels of this immunoglobulin.

3.3. Genetic factors in the synthesis and control of the immunoglobulins

A knowledge of the anatomy of the immunoglobulins allows us now to consider a genetic model to explain the variations that are observed. As in the description of the molecule, we will start with a simple genetic model envisaging restricted variation, and then amplify it until all the known variation in the structure of these proteins is covered.

At first it seemed, although highly unlikely, that the immunoglobulins were single gene products, the resultant polypeptides being broken up into two fragments, heavy and light chains. In fact, in 1944 Beadle and Tatum proposed the theory that each protein of micro-organisms and multicellular organisms was the product of a single gene. But this is certainly not the case here. The simplest possibility would be the existence of two genes, one for the heavy and another for the light chain. This minimal model would perhaps be acceptable if there were only a single class of immunoglobulins, but as there are five known classes, there need to be at least five genes for the heavy chains. Similarly, to account for the two classes of light chains, a gene for the $\varkappa$ chain and a gene for the λ chain need to be postulated. There are however four different classes of γ chain, two of α and two of μ chains, so there must be genes coding for at least four γ, two α and two μ chains, and one each for the δ and ε chains. Thus some 12 genes are required.

The hypothesis of two genes, one polypeptide

Based on the structure of Bence–Jones proteins and L chains from mouse myelomas, Dreyer and Bennett suggested in 1965 that two genes, instead of one, were involved in the synthesis of each immunoglobulin chain. Almost simultaneously, other investigators engaged in sequencing human Bence–Jones proteins found that the constant region was always the same within a given type of L chain, but that they all differ in their variable regions. These results gave support to the theory of two genes, one polypeptide. The amino acid studies of the H chain also indicated that here too there were two genes, coding for the C and V regions. Moreover, the five subgroups of V regions in the heavy chains are not exclusive to any one of the classes or subclasses of immunoglobulins. Finally, even clearer evidence came from Fudenberg's studies. Analysing a human serum with two monoclonal proteins (IgG2 and IgM) he found that the γ and μ chains differed in their C regions but were very similar in their V regions. Family studies in this patient showed clearly the presence of two genes. Other data from this patient are also relevant. By immunofluorescent techniques it was shown that different cells synthesize the two C regions and the same V region. As a consequence, Fudenberg proposed the existence of a switch mechanism that stops the production of the C region of the μ chain and starts that of the C region of the γ chain. Other laboratories have extended the observations to IgA (see p. 28).

Returning then to our genetic model, if each H and L chain is coded for by two genes, we need to double our estimate and add at least five more genes for the V_H subgroups so far identified. Similarly, four V-region subgroups are known for the $\varkappa$ chains and six for the λ chains, but again the final numbers are not yet established. Altogether therefore we must postulate some 15 genes coding for V regions and another 15 for C regions. Yet the problem is far more complicated.

Recombinant DNA techniques

Once recombinant DNA methods became available a few years ago, a clearer picture of immunoglobulin genetics emerged by the characterization of the immunoglobulin genes. These techniques allow any DNA sequence to be inserted into a plasmid or phage and then propagated. Usually, the isolation of the desired gene requires the assembly and screening of a DNA library, which may be genomic if it contains all the sequences in the genome irrespective of their coding capability, or a cDNA library if it is a synthesized double-stranded copy of the mRNA. Once the gene-specific probe (the desired gene) has been identified, a Southern blotting is usually performed. This procedure consists of cleaving a random nucleotide sequence into thousands of small fragments by means of a restriction endonuclease. The detection of specific classes of sequences within these is obtained by blotting (hence the name) these fragments on to nitrocellulose after separating them by gel electrophoresis according to their molecular weight. Once on the nitrocellulose, they are incubated with the ^{32}P-labelled sequence probe which will hybridize to its complement. After the unhybridized DNA has been washed away, the position of the hybridization on the nitrocellulose is detected by autoradiography.

This technique has shown that multiple gene segments in the germ-line cells encode the component immunoglobulin polypeptides, which join together to form an active immunoglobulin in the B cell.

The mouse immunoglobulin genes

Mouse immunoglobulins are encoded by three unlinked groups of genes: λ (chromosome 16), ϰ (chromosome 6) and heavy (H) chain genes (chromosome 12).

The lambda chain is coded for by three DNA segments: V, J and C. Starting from the 5′ end of the nucleotide sequence, there is a precursor or leading sequence (L) separated from the V segment by an intervening sequence of around 100 base pairs (bp) long (in fact, part of the L sequence is coded for by the V sequence as well). There is then another intervening sequence of unknown length between the V and J segments and still another of around 1000 bp long between the J and C segments at the 3′ end (Figure 3.3). In those cells which express the lambda gene, the V and J sequences are fused without the intervening sequence. The V sequence codes for most of the variable region of the light chain except the FR₄ which is coded for by the J segment. The C sequence codes obviously for the total C peptide. This lambda-chain system in the mouse, with only three J–C segments and two L–V segments, is not very variable.

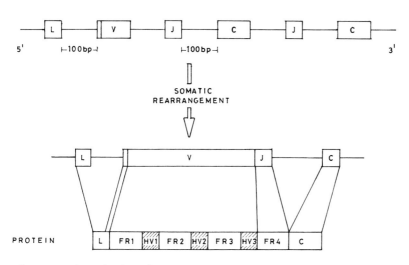

Figure 3.3. Organization of the lambda chain and genes.

The kappa gene segments show a similar but much more variable constitution. The haploid genome contains a single copy of a C_k segment, five different J_k segments and between 100 and 500 V_k segments, each with its preceding leader sequence.

In the heavy chains the haploid germ line contains between 100 and 200 L_H-V_H segments, 12 D and four J segments and eight copies of the C_H segment corresponding to the classes and subclasses of immunoglobulins. It is worth noting that each one of the C_H segments is made up of various coding sequences (exons) which correspond to the structural domains of the immunoglobulin.

The human immunoglobulin genes

The human immunoglobulin genes are also basically controlled by three unlinked gene clusters: λ (chromosome 22), κ (chromosome 2) and heavy-chain genes (chromosome 14). The general distribution of these genetic segments is similar to those of the mouse. The V_k and V_H both have at the 5′ end a leader sequence of around 20 bp length and a short intervening sequence, similar to that of the mouse, which divides the signal peptide into two pieces.

The V gene segments are uninterrupted and similar in the V_H and V_k, except that in the latter the CDR_3 is encoded within the V segment itself, while in the heavy-chain genes the CDR_3 sequence is found outside the V region (D sequence). The total number of V genes seems to be much smaller in man than in mice. In fact, it is calculated that in man there are only about 20–30 V_k genes, and a similar number of V_H segments.

The human V_λ gene repertoire is larger than that of the mouse. The human lambda constant region consists of at least four non-allelic forms that differ by limited amino acid substitutions to produce the serological markers Kern, Oz and Mcg. Several additional λ variants have been identified, but it is not known whether they represent allelic variants or different isotypes. The lambda constant region genes are six in number, located in a 30 kb (kb = kilobase = 1000 bases) segment (Figure 3.3). Three of them correspond to three of the four known allelic variants of lambda C genes. One of the other three is presumably the $Ke^+ Oz^-$. More recently it has been observed that the human lambda immunoglobulin locus displays a series of restriction fragment length polymorphisms, presumably arising from unequal crossing-over between $Ke^- Oz^-$ and $Ke^- Oz^+$. It has been suggested therefore that this unequal meiotic crossing-over may alter the number of λ genes from six to nine, introducing more capacity for variation to the λ light-chain genes.

3.4. Assembly of the immunoglobulin genes

So far we have described the position of the various immunoglobulin genes within the genome of the germ-line cell, but there is a fairly complex process of reorganization of the products of these genes to complete the formation of each immunoglobulin molecule.

Joining signals

The mechanisms that induce the joining of the V, J and C gene products are unknown. However, it has been observed that there are repetitive sequences in the introns between the V and J segments that may act as joining signals. The segments so far studied (V_k, V_λ, V_H and D) in mouse and man have shown that downstream (from 5′ to 3′) from the V genes there are two sequences of 7 and 9 bases (CACAGTC and ACAAAAACC) separated by a spacer 12 or 23 bp long. A similar insertion is observed between the D and J segments. There is also a report of the identification of a short region in the intron between the human J_k and C_k genes, neither translated nor independently transcribed, which may have a regulatory role as an enhancer element. This region has been provisionally named kappa intron conserved region (KICR).

The joining of the C, V and J segments probably occurs in two steps, one of them at the DNA level and the other at the mRNA level. At the DNA level and during the differentiation process, the larger intervening sequence between V and J is lost, leaving together the J and V sequences. During the synthesis of the mRNA in the B cell, the other intervening sequence between J and C is lost together with the spare C and V genes, leaving only one of each C, V and J sequences joined together and ready for the synthesis of the protein.

Intracodonal J–V joining

The end-point of the immunoglobulin gene segments is not precise. In kappa chains, for instance, the V_k gene usually ends at the position corresponding to amino acid number 95 and the beginning of the J_k gene corresponds to amino acid 96. However, this is not always the case, and the V–J joining may take place one or two nucleotides downstream of codon 95 leading to the presence of different codons for amino acid 96. Since this amino acid forms part of the CDR3, it has been argued that this mechanism may well play a role in generating more antibody diversity. Still further variation may come from free insertion of a few nucleotides at the VH–D and C–JH junctions.

3.5. The expression of immunoglobulin genes during development

As mentioned in Chapter 2, during the latter part of the maturation of the B lymphocyte there may occur the sequential expression of the immunoglobulin genes.

In the B-cell precursor, the recombination and activation of the μ-chain genes precedes that of the light chains. In fact, pre-B cells express cytoplasmic μ chains before light or other heavy chains are expressed. There are however two distinct forms of μ-chain synthesis in B cells: membrane and secretory μ chains, the former being larger and hydrophobic.

In a single B cell, only the Ig genes of a single chromosome of the available pair are used in the heavy- and light-chain synthesis. This phenomenon is called allelic exclusion. There is also isotype exclusion since the cell has to select between the λ and $\varkappa$ gene expression. In the former process immature B lymphocytes assemble and express only membrane IgM, then with further maturation another rearrangement occurs, expressing in the cell a different C_H gene with the same V_H, V_L and C_L. This is known as 'class switch', and allows the generation of antibodies which are functionally diverse but with identical specificity. It seems that the mechanism by which this class switching is obtained is a process of looping and deletion. In the germ-line DNA the human heavy-chain genes are located from 5' to 3' as follows: $C\mu$, $C\delta$, $C\gamma$, $C\varepsilon$, $C\alpha$. When the variable D and J segments are to join a $C\gamma$, for instance, there is a looping out and deletion of the sequence containing the $C\mu$ and $C\delta$ genes. The majority of splenic lymphocytes bear both IgD and IgM simultaneously in their membranes. This results from the splicing in of two different forms, a single mRNA that contains the V_H, D, J_H and both $C\mu$ and $C\delta$. The co-expression of this double isotype is lost during the differentiation towards cells expressing either IgG or IgA.

Quality control

Besides these various mechanisms to account for antibody diversity, it is also necessary to account for the functionality of the end-product, that is the immunoglobulin. It seems clear that there is no genetic mechanism restricted to the production of functional antibody molecules only, and hence if not all the molecules produced are functional, it is necessary to explain the way in which elimination occurs of the genes that code for non-functional molecules, and how those that produce molecules of optimal quality are selected.

Two mechanisms have been proposed. Cohn suggested that the antibodies that do not combine with antigen are selected against by an unspecified mechanism that eliminates cells which have not responded to antigenic stimulation during a given period of time. In the alternative proposal, Jerne suggests that antibodies of varied specificity are obtained by mutation affecting their affinity for histocompatibility antigens, and selection would then be based on the retention of anti-self activity. There are as yet insufficient data to decide which of these mechanisms is responsible for the elimination of unnecessary antibodies.

3.6. Genetic markers of the immunoglobulins

As the name indicates, the genetic markers allow the identification of the genetic mechanisms involved in the synthesis of the immunoglobulin molecule, and although it was initially thought that they were not of much importance in the antigenic heterogeneity expressed by the individual, recent observations suggest that they may play an important role in determining disease susceptibility (see Chapter 11). Most of the information so far summarized about the immunoglobulins has been obtained with the help of these markers, called allotypes, that are found in humans as in every vertebrate that possesses an immune system.

Five sets of allotypes have been described for human immunoglobulins. Four are present in heavy chains and are called Gm, Am, Mm and Em, and one is present only in the $\varkappa$ type of light chain, today called Km and previously known as Inv. The nomenclature used for these allotypes consist of letters indicating the class of chain (Gm, Mm, etc.), a number which indicates a specific subclass (e.g., G1m, A2m), followed by a number in brackets that shows the allotypic determinant (e.g., G1m(1), G1m(17)). The alleles in each system are expressed as numbers, and sometimes letters, to the right of the letter that designates the corresponding marker, for example Gm^1 or Am^2. The W.H.O. recommended nomenclature for the known allotypic markers is shown in Table 3.2, together with the old designation in order to avoid confusion.

What the allotypic markers are in chemical terms is less easy to answer than where they are located in the structure of the immunoglobulin molecule. The Km factors are only present in light chains of the $\varkappa$ type, and so can be found in all five classes of immunoglobulin. The Gm, Am and Mm markers are found in the heavy chains of the IgG, IgA and IgM molecules, respectively. Except for the two factors(G1m(4) and G1m(17)) that are located on the Fab fragment, all the Gm markers are in the Fc region of the γ chains. A correlation has been demonstrated between Gm markers and the IgG subclasses. As can be seen in Table 3.2, G1m(4), (1), (2) and (17) are found only on the IgG1 subclass, while only one marker has been found on IgG2 (G2m(23)) and several on IgG3.

So far we have given an idea of the location of the genetic and allotypic markers on the immunoglobulins. Let us now see what this means in structural terms. The variations which explain the allotypes of the immunoglobulins are derived from several factors, for example, from changes in the amino acid sequence of the chain, or from its content of carbohydrates, or from a combination of both. Amino acid studies have proved that the Km and the majority of the Gm markers derive from changes in the amino acid sequences of the chain. In greater detail, the three allotypic determinants of the Km system, which are localized in the constant region of the type $\varkappa$ chains, depend on changes at two positions, 153 and 191. The allotypic determinant Km(1) has valine and leucine at these positions, Km(1;2) has alanine and leucine, and Km(3) has alanine and valine. No other difference has been observed between the allotypic determinants of the Km system.

For the markers of the Gm system the situation is similar but more complicated, as in this case the changes are not in one but in several adjacent amino acids. For example, the study of the chains of IgG shows that the peptides are different when the protein is typified or not typified as G1m(1). Studies of the sequencing of these two polypeptides show differences in the residues 356–360. When the protein is G1m(1) these positions are occupied by the amino acids Asp-Glu-Leu-

Human immunogenetics

Table 3.2. Some allotypes of human immunoglobulins

Allotypes	Allotypic markers	
	Letters	Numbers (WHO)
IgG1		
G1m	a	1
	x	2
	f,bw or b2	3 or 4
	z	17
IgG2		
G2m	n	23
IgG3		
G3m	b0	11
	b1	5
	b3	13
	b4	14
	b5	10
	c3,like	6
	c5	24
	g	21
	s	15
	t	16
	u	26
	v	27
IgA2		1
A2m		2
k Chain		
Km		1
		2
		3

Thr-Lys and when the protein is negative for the G1m(1) allotype these positions are occupied by the amino acids Glu-Glu-Met-Thr-Lys. Such changes appear to be those responsible for determining the allotypes of the Gm system.

In the same way have been found amino acid substitutions associated with G1m(4), G3m(5) and G3m(21). The nature of the genetic markers of IgA2 have not been established, but the absence of H–L disulphide bonds in the A2m(1) chains suggests that there has been some substitution of amino acids in this case.

Inheritance of all these systems is very similar. The Km system has three allotypic determinants *Km(1)*, *Km(2)* and *Km(3)*, controlled by a single locus with three codominant alleles, Km^1, $Km^{1,2}$ and Km^3. The two markers that have been described for IgA2 are allelic forms which determine A2m(1) and A2m(2).

The inheritance of the Gm factors is similar but rather more complicated, since they are not inherited individually but in haplotypes, which behave like codominant alleles similar to the Km and Am systems. These haplotypes are not clearly constant but vary in frequency from one population to another, and particular variants are associated with specific populations.

Reflections on antibody diversity

The models summarized in this chapter of the genetic mechanisms involved in the synthesis of immunoglobulins have contributed much towards a better understanding of the generation of diversity, but have not solved the philosophical questions behind it. There has been much argument about whether all antibody diversity is completely genetically controlled or is induced by the cellular environment. It is therefore reassuring to know that part of it can be explained in terms of rearrangement of inherited gene sequences. There is still however some variation, the so-called somatic diversifiers (imprecise joining ends and free insertion of nucleotides), whose molecular mechanisms are as yet unknown. They too may be controlled by a genetic mechanism (e.g., by some signal within the genome), but it is also possible that the antigen itself plays a role in their induction. Perhaps a second messenger type of signal takes the information from cell membrane to the nucleus, but even then there is an information gap. After all, genetic as well as computer languages are written at different levels: cells speak machine language (DNA) and hence it seems difficult to feed them with information from the environment, unless there is something like an assembler program carrying out the conversion of this information into DNA sequences. The problem is that an assembler, being a program itself, has to be written in some compatible language, somewhere. How and where is it done in the cell?

3.7. Genetic control of the immunoglobulin levels

Besides the genetic control at the structural level discovered recently, there has been investigation of the genetic control of immunoglobulin levels, the resultant of the rates of synthesis and catabolism. The problem has been approached in five different ways.

Animal models have been used to study the associations between immunoglobulin levels and the chromosome complement. Twin and family studies have been more appropriate for obtaining heritability estimates. In this type of study the immunoglobulin levels show a low to moderate heritability. Family studies also allow the following of a given trait in successive generations (for instance the low levels of an immunoglobulin). In these cases the genetic effects are more clear cut, particularly for low levels of IgD and IgE which have been shown to be inherited in a straight Mendelian form, suggesting the effect of a single functional locus. The study of isolated or combined immunodeficiencies has also been rewarding, since many of these defects show a clear pattern of inheritance. Finally, population studies have given information regarding the associations between immunoglobulin levels and genetic markers. The various reports using this type of approach record associations between the IgG levels and the Lewis blood groups, secretor, haptoglobin types and the ABO blood groups, and between IgA and 6-phosphoglucodehydrogenase (6PGD) types. Our own experience in this respect is rather contradictory, for these associations were not found consistently in a large series of various ethnic groups. Nevertheless, our study shows other interesting features like the correlations between the levels of the different immunoglobulins themselves. A point not yet clear in this respect is whether the genes affecting the levels of one immunoglobulin may also affect those of others. In animal studies it has been possible to cross mice to produce high or low levels of IgG and IgM. Moreover, it has been shown that mice responding with high levels of IgE to a given antigen also respond with high levels of IgG to the same antigen. These results suggest the probable presence of a common mechanism of genetic control for several of the immunoglobulin levels in mice.

Our population studies in man show a similar feature, since it was found that populations with high environmental stress maintain high IgG and IgE levels and a relative diminution of IgA (Figure 3.4), suggesting also a common control of immunoglobulin levels particularly for IgG, IgA and IgM.

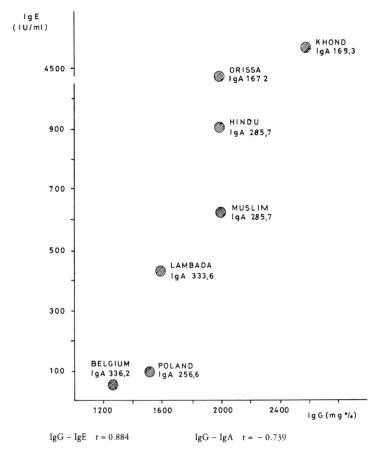

Figure 3.4. Levels of IgG, IgA and IgE in various populations showing their interrelationship.

Other interesting aspects of the genetic control of the levels of these proteins relate to their association with the HLA system and the immunoglobulin allotypes. The total levels of IgG do not seem to be affected by the Gm markers but the IgG subclasses are. The levels of IgG3 are for instance twice as high in homozygous G3m(5) as in homozygous G3m(21). For IgG2 a similar situation has been observed, since individuals' G2m(23) have very high levels of IgG4 although this subclass has no allotypes. A more recent report also associates the low levels of IgE and IgD with the markers G1m(3) and G3m(5). As regards the HLA system, low levels of IgE have been observed associated with HLA-A2 in normal Icelandic families, and we have observed an association between low IgM levels and HLA-B12 in patients and families with spinal muscular atrophy.

3.8. The evolution of the immunoglobulins

The synthesis of specific antibodies is an immunological property of the vertebrates, while cellular immunity is present in lower life forms. Of all the immunoglobulins IgM may have been the first to appear in the evolution of the immune system, by a process of gene duplication from a primordial gene that coded for one of what are today known as domains. It is possible that this genetic duplication was attained first by a tandem duplication, in which a DNA segment is totally or partially duplicated, and later by a combination of tandem and

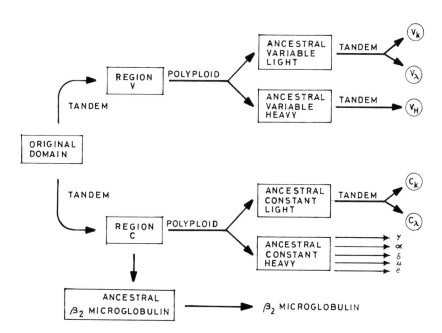

Figure 3.5. Diagram of the possible evolution of immunoglobulins.

polyploid duplications (Figure 3.5). This evolutionary process can be summarized in three steps:

1. Formation of the variable and constant regions of heavy and light chains.
2. Formation of the various classes of heavy and light chains.
3. Formation of subclasses and subtypes.

These mechanisms, although still hypothetical, are supported by the studies of amino acid sequencing of the immunoglobulins. For instance, when the sequence of the V and C regions of the heavy and light chains is observed, certain similarities are apparent, particularly in size and position of disulphide bridges. The similarities suggest that V and C regions come from a common ancestor, but diverged very early in the evolution of the immune system. On the other hand, the similarity between the constant regions of heavy and light genes is very marked, suggesting that the duplication of the ancestral gene gave as a first result both the C regions of the heavy and light chains, and then a later duplication of the heavy-chain gene produced a heavy chain twice the size of the light chain.

Evolution of the heavy-chain classes

It seems that IgG and IgA evolved from IgM. It is known that the heavy chain of IgM has one domain more than IgA and IgG. If this domain is not considered homologous to the hinge region, it is possible that the loss of the $C\mu2$ domain led to the formation of the γ chain while the loss of the $C\mu$ domain led to the formation of the α chain. The ε chain may have arisen as a tandem duplication of the IgM gene. These suggestions will certainly change as a result of the direct genetic analysis of these genes by means of restriction DNA technology.

Allotypes

The formation of allotypes as well as of the γ subclasses seems to have been a more recent evolutionary event and, as a result, the majority of the Gm markers are confined to a single γ subclass.

Timescale of immune evolution

If it is assumed that two genes coming from a common ancestor differentiated at a constant rate, it is possible to calculate the time that has elapsed since their differentiation by the study of their products in species descended from common ancestors. In other words, the number of base-pair differences between two genes is proportional to the time since their origin in the common ancestor. These rates are calculated in amino acid residues per chain per million years, and it has been observed that each type of chain has its own rate. Haemoglobin, for instance, has a rate of 0.14 residues per chain per million years. These studies, so far limited, have shown that for the immunoglobulins the rate is slightly higher, about 0.2 residues per chain per million years.

Comparing these differences, and more recently comparing gene maps, it has been suggested that the separation of the μ and γ chains took place some 200 million years ago and the divergence of the γ chain subclasses occurred 20–30 million years ago. The expansion of the J_k cluster of genes is a much more recent event, only one or two million years ago. In view of the great length of time that it has taken to evolve the efficient immune system that is man's today, one wonders if any possible improvement could be attained by somatic mutation, which can only be random, during the development of a single individual (see p. 31).

Bibliography

Bazaral, M., Orgel, H. A. and Hamburger, R. N., Genetics of IgE and allergy: serum IgE levels in twins. *J. Allergy Clin. Immunol.*, **54**: 288 (1974).

Billewicz, W. Z., McGregor, I. A., Roberts, D. F. and Rowe, D. S., Family studies of immunoglobulin levels. *Clin. Exp. Immunol.*, **16**: 13 (1974).

Burnet, F. M., *The Production of Antibodies*. MacMillan, Melbourne (1941).

Burstein, Y., Breiner, A. V., Brandt, C. E., Milcarek, C., Sweet, R. W., Warszawski, D., Ziv, E. and Schechter, I., Recent duplication and germ-line diversification of rat immunoglobulin *x* chain gene joining segments. *Proc. Natl. Acad. Sci. USA.*, **79**: 5993 (1982).

Charke, S. H., Claflin, J. L. and Rudikoff, S., Polymorphisms in immunoglobulin heavy chains suggesting gene conversion. *Proc. Natl. Acad. Sci. USA*, **79**: 3280 (1982).

Coleclough, C., Chance, necessity and antibody gene dynamics. *Nature*, **303**: 23 (1983).

Dreyer, W. J. and Bennett, J. C., The molecular basis of antibody formation: a paradox. *Proc. Natl. Acad. Sci. USA*, **54**: 864 (1965).

Dunette, S. L., Gleich, G. J. and Weinshilboum, R. M., Inheritance of low serum immuno-globulin D. *J. Clin. Invest.*, **62**: 248 (1978).

Edelman, G. M. and Gally, J. A., Somatic recombination of duplicated genes: an hypothesis on the origin of antibody diversity. *Proc. Natl. Acad. Sci. USA*, **57**: 353 (1967).

Fahey, J. L., Antibodies and immunoglobulins. Structure and function. *J.A.M.A.*, **194**: (1965).

Giblett, E. R., *Genetic Markers in Human Blood*. F. A. Davis, Philadelphia (1969).

Grubb, R., *The Genetic Markers of Human Immunoglobulins*. Springer-Verlag, New York (1970).

Grundbacher, F. J. and Shreffler, D. C., Effects of secretor, blood and serum groups on isoantibody and immunoglobulin levels. *Am. J. Hum. Genet.*, **22**: 194 (1970).

Hill, R. L., Delaney, R., Fellows, R. E. and Lebovitz, H. E., The evolutionary origins of the immunoglobulins. *Proc. Natl. Acad. Sci. USA*, **56**: 1792 (1966).

Hobbs, J. R., Immunoglobulins. *Clin. Chem.*, **14**: 220 (1972).

Hood, L. and Talmage, D. W., Mechanisms of antibody diversity; germ line basis for variability. *Science*, **168**: 325 (1970).

Leder, P., The genetics of antibody diversity. *Sci. Am.*, **246**: 72 (1982).

Nahar, R. A., Bernal, J. E. and Wolanski, N., Serum immunoglobulin levels and genetic polymorphism: a study in Poland. *J. Hum. Evol.*, **11**: 721 (1982).

Natvig, J. B. and Kunkel, H. G., Human immunoglobulins: classes, subclasses, genetic variants and idiotypes. *Adv. Immunol.*, **16**: 1 (1973).

Roberts, D. F., Al-Agidi, S. K. and Vincent, K., Immunoglobulin levels and genetic polymorphisms in the Sukuma of Tanzania. *Ann. Hum. Biol.*, **6**: 105 (1979).

Taub, R. A., Hollis, G. F., Hieter, P. A., Korsmeyer, S., Waldmann, T. A. and Leder, P., Variable amplification of immunoglobulin and light-chain genes in human populations. *Nature*, **304**: 172 (1983).

Tomasi, T. B. and Grey, H. M., Structure and function of immunoglobulin A., *Prog. Allergy*, **16**: 81 (1972).

Van Lozhem, E., The immunoglobulin genes: genetics, biological and clinical significance. *Clin. Immunol. Allergy*, **4**(3): 3607 (1984).

Wood, G. B. S., Martin, W., Adinolfi, M. and Polani, P. E., Immunoglobulins and the X-chromosome. *Br. Med. J.*, **4**: 110 (1969).

Chapter 4. The major histocompatibility system

In the immune response cellular interaction takes place in two ways: through a series of surface antigens, and through the secretion of some products, of which the best known are the immunoglobulins produced by the plasma cells. There are very many antigens or markers on the cell surface. One group of them forms a system, the subject of this chapter, that involves many genetic loci and that has been identified in every vertebrate species so far studied. The products of these genes participate in a variety of immune functions, and this 'knot' of linked genes is known as the major histocompatibility system (MHS) or complex (MHC). The MHS has different names in different species: RT1 in the rat, DLA in the dog, H-2 in the mouse and HLA in man. Here only the most important aspects of the H-2, which has contributed so much to basic understanding of histocompatibility, and HLA will be reviewed, but in sufficient detail to provide a clear picture of their scientific and clinical importance.

4.1. The H-2 system

The total number of genes in the major histocompatibility system of the mouse is not known, but may run into several hundred. The H-2 genes are located on chromosome 17, and by means of recombination studies the relevant section of it has been divided into six regions, designated as K, I, S, D, L and R. These studies have allowed two important features of the MHS to be established: the genetic map, and the number of genes involved in the immune response to certain antigens. The frequency with which two genes recombine is directly related to the distance between them. The further apart they are, the greater the probability that they will recombine. Figure 4.1 shows the genetic map of the H-2 system. From it, one would expect the recombination frequency to be higher between the K and D regions, for instance, than between the K and I, and this is in fact what happens; the observed recombination frequency between the former is about 0.2%, while between the latter it is 0.03%. In the genetic map these results are

37

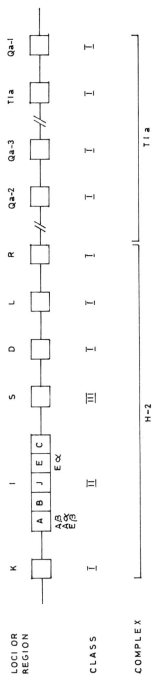

Figure 4.1. The major histocompatibility complex (H-2) on chromosome 17 of the mouse.

expressed in units of centimorgans (cM), 1% recombination frequency being equivalent to one centimorgan or about 2000 kb. By these recombination frequencies the position of the genes illustrated in Figure 4.1 was established.

Recombination studies have also been used to examine the number of genes involved in the response to different antigens. For example if the immune response to two different antigens is controlled by a single gene, the crossing of animals with and without that gene will give offspring that respond either to both or none, but no offspring responding to only one of them. Since both responses are controlled by a single gene, recombination (except at the intragene level) is impossible. If, on the other hand, the responses to the two antigens are controlled by two separate but linked genes, one would expect that most progeny would respond to both or neither and occasionally by recombination to one or the other. This type of manipulation has been used in the preparation of strains of congenic animals that differ in only one of the regions of the MHS, allowing antibodies to be obtained that are specific for only one of those regions. Every one of the H-2 regions, except the S region, controls the expression of a series of membrane proteins. These can be grouped into three types: the antigenic specificities under the control of K, D, L and R regions (class I), the Ia specificities depending on the I region (class II), and the class III which are serum components of the complement system.

K and D regions

These regions are functionally as well as structurally related, and it has been suggested that both evolved by tandem duplication from a common ancestral gene. As regards the function of these two products, it has been observed in viral specific cytotoxic reactions that they behave as adaptors, binding viral antigens and forming a complex that can be recognized by a special subgroup of T cells. They also control the response against the Thy-1 antigen, stimulate the production of a soluble factor that helps the final maturation of B cells, and their determinants play a role in the mixed-lymphocyte culture and the graft-versus-host reaction.

Private and public specificities

Each allele of the K and D regions controls or determines the expression of a set of antigenic determinants, of which only one is characteristic of that allele and is not controlled by any other allele. A specificity of this type is called private. The other antigenic determinants of that set are also present in the sets of other alleles of the same or even different regions. These are therefore known as public specificities. If one of these public specificities is present in the set of several alleles, it is said to be a broad public specificity, otherwise it will be narrow. Public specificities can also be classified according to the regions involved in uni- or bi-regional categories, if the alleles that determine them are in one or in several regions.

S region

This region controls the quantitative levels of the Ss protein that is the equivalent of the C4 of human complement. Some alleles have been defined, and at least four of them are characterized by high levels of this protein. The Slp locus is also in this region and controls the expression of the 'sex-limited protein', a homologue of the fourth component of murine complement. Both C4 and Slp are synthesized as antigenically distinct single-chain precursors of molecular weight around 20 000, subsequently cleaved into the α, β and γ chains. The Slp protein has no haemolytic activity.

I region

At least five subregions are known within this region, named I-A, I-B, I-C, I-E and I-J. The immune response genes (Ir genes) to certain antigens are found in this region, and their products in the cell membrane are known as immune-associated or Ia antigens, and occur on the cell surface of most B lymphocytes, macrophages and some other cells including a T-lymphocyte subpopulation. About 20 Ia-specific monoclonal antibodies have been reported.

A second family of I-region gene products has recently been found, and called the Iat molecules. These are present on some T lymphocytes and regulatory T-cell products but not on B lymphocytes. The first of these molecules, Iat.W40, is a specificity of the I-J^k subregion, characteristic of mature peripheral T cells but absent from thymocytes. A second Iat molecule, Iat.W46, is controlled by a gene which maps between the I-J and I-E subregions, and finally a third Iat antigen, Iat.W41 (the Ia-7 locus), maps between H-2k and Ia.

The Ia antigens play various roles in the immune system, and are particularly essential in antigen recognition by T lymphocytes involved in proliferation, helper functions and delayed hypersensitivity. The process of antigen recognition by the T cells sometimes requires the presentation of the antigen in association with an Ia molecule on the surface of an accessory cell, resulting in the so-called H-2 restriction mechanism. The precise molecular mechanism involved in the action of the Ia molecules is unknown. Nevertheless, there is abundant evidence to show that the expression of Ia determinants on the surface of the macrophage is required for effective presentation of the antigen by the macrophage to T cells. The restriction mechanism is not confined to Ia (class II) antigens. Helper T cells and those responsible for delayed hypersensitivity recognize class II antigens, but cytotoxic T cells use class I antigens. There is also evidence suggesting that there is an active interaction between the antigen and the Ia determinant on the surface of the macrophage, but its nature is unknown.

The structure of the T-cell receptor is still largely unknown, and so it is not possible to say whether it recognizes the antigen and the MHC determinant as two separate entities (the dual recognition theory) or as a single 'neoantigen' created by the combination of antigen and MHC determinant (altered-self theory). Other functions of the I region are the genetic control of specific immune responses, discussed in further detail later, but which map mainly within the I-A subregion; the suppression of immune responses through what have been called immune suppressor genes (Is); and also control of strong antigenic determinants both as activators of the mixed-lymphocyte-culture reaction as well as transplantation antigens.

Of the known subregions of the I region, the I-A and I-E are well studied. The I-J seems to encode soluble T-cell factors and cell-surface antigens on T cells and macrophages not yet characterized, while the I-B and I-C regions are in limbo, defined only on their apparent control of certain immune responses.

4.2. Molecular structure of the H-2 antigens

Class I antigens

These antigens are made up of two proteins: one, very polymorphic, of molecular weight around 45 000 and a smaller peptide, of molecular weight 12 000, called β2-microglobulin. The heavier chain is a glycoprotein and has a transmembrane disposition on the cell surface, with part of it exposed to the cytoplasm. Like the arrangement seen in the immunoglobulins, these products have domains, a total of five in the heavy chain. Three of them are outside the cell membrane, and two smaller ones are located within the cell membrane and in the cytoplasm. The external domains are called α1 (the amino terminal), α2 and α3. The total heavy chain contains some 350 amino acids, 90 in each of the external domains plus 30 in each of the other two domains.

The light chain, β2-microglobulin, has only 99 amino acids in mouse and 100 in man, and is not encoded within the major histocompatibility complex but in a different chromosome (2 in mouse, 15 in man). By amino acid sequencing there has been observed a marked homology between the β2-microglobulin and the constant regions of the x, λ and H chains of the immunoglobulins, and more recently also to the α3 domain of the class I antigens. This similarity is also observed at the functional level since β2-microglobulin is capable, for instance, of fixing complement. It has been suggested therefore that the gene coding for the β2-microglobulin may be the product of a duplication of one of the ancestor genes of the immunoglobulins. On the cell surface, the β2-microglobulin binds the α3 domain of the class I antigens.

Class II antigens

These antigens consist of three protein chains, called α, β and γ, the first two with similar molecular weights (33 000 and 28 000, respectively). Each of the α and β chains has four domains: two outside the cell, one transmembrane and one cytoplasmic. Little is known about the third chain, but it has been recently observed that as the class I antigens need the β2 microglobulin for their expression and function, the class II antigens require a polypeptide known as invariant chain (Ii) which is only associated with the intracellular but not the cell-surface form of these products. Ii, which is coded for by a gene not linked to the H-2, may play a role in the assembly or intracellular transport of the class II antigens.

As regards polymorphism, both the α and β chains vary from molecule to molecule, but it seems that class II antigens are overall less polymorphic than the class I antigens. It has been calculated that there may be up to 60 alleles at each one of the loci of class I antigens but only 10–15 variants for some of the class II antigens.

The molecular map of the H-2

DNA technology is also proving of benefit in mapping the H-2 system. Recently it has shown that the I-A and I-E subregions seem to be separated by a segment of DNA of less than 1000 bases which is not enough for encoding the I-B and I-J regions. Therefore, it has been suggested that at least the I-J product may be encoded outside the I region. So far a map has been obtained of the region comprising the segments coding for the α and β chains of the I-A and I-E products. The order of these genes seems to be: centromere–$A\alpha$–$A\beta$–$E\beta$ and $E\alpha$. A second $E\beta$ sequence was also identified between the $E\beta$ and $E\alpha$ that may be either a pseudogene or a functional gene so far serologically unidentified. The $A\alpha$, $A\beta$ and $E\beta$ chains are encoded in the I-A subregion whereas the $E\alpha$ is encoded in the I-E subregion. This means that while the totality of the I-A product is coded for by exons within the I-A region, the I-E product is coded for by an exon in its own region (the α chain) and another in the I-A region (the β chain). This mechanism has been called complementation by linked genes. It is likely therefore that as new probes become available they will change our view of the I region even more; some of the old regions will disappear while new functional segments will be revealed which were not discovered by the older immunological methods. Perhaps the important point to bear in mind is that so far the map of the MHC has been drawn by means of recombinational events of identified products and functions, but some of these products may not be the results of a single gene and some of the functions may be performed by more than one product.

As with the immunoglobulins, there is a correspondence between the protein domains and the distribution of introns and exons in the genomic DNA sequence of the H-2 antigen. After a leader sequence, the genomic DNA of a class I antigen has three coding sequences separated by introns, then the transmembrane sequence, followed by three exons coding for the cytoplasmic portion. Class II antigen genes are similar; after the leader sequence there are two exons coding for the domains $\alpha 1$ and $\alpha 2$, and another two exons code for the transmembrane and cytoplasmic portions plus the 3′ untranslated region.

4.3. Polymorphism at the major histocompatibility complex

It has already been mentioned that both α and β chains are polymorphic, but more markedly in class I antigens. Analysis of the heavy-chain sequences as well as their cloned genes have shown that the differences between the various genes are not confined to single-base changes but to changes in short sequences of the DNA. Almost all of these 'clusters' have been found in the two most external domains of the proteins; the largest and most complex so far described is that of the class I antigens of BALB/C mouse, with 13 gene clusters containing 36 distinct class I genes and encompassing 837 kb of DNA. Thirty-one of these map within the Tla, Qa regions. More intriguing still is the finding of a marked homology between the genes at different loci. It has been calculated that the homology between alleles is $\cong 90\%$ in terms of amino acid identity, while that among genes of different loci is about 85%.

Various mechanisms have been suggested to explain this high degree of homologous diversity. At first it was thought that the alleles may not be alleles of a single gene but rather a linked group of different genes. This has been shown not to be the case. Another possibility is unequal crossing over due to misalignment of two genes on homologous chromosomes during meiosis. It is possible that this process accounts for part of the diversity, but more attention has been given recently to a very attractive hypothesis — gene conversion. This mechanism, originally described in fungi, allows the transference of genetic information from one gene to another related gene anywhere in the genome, although it is more frequent between alleles. The underlying genetic mechanism of gene conversion is not well understood, but is is probably due to pairing between sequences in part homologous during meiosis, followed by mis-match repair.

If this is the mechanism at work in the creation of diversity within the MHC, the observed clusters of genes would be the result of gene conversion, and it should then be possible to find the original genes from which these sequences come. Some investigators have indeed succeeded in finding a potential donor for a mutant heavy chain among a library of some 90 clones of class I antigens. It is rather interesting that this and other potential donors seem to map within the Tla, Qa region, next to the H-2, and are con..dered by some as part of the major histocompatibility complex (see below).

Besides the sequence homology of class I antigens, two other features support the existence of gene conversion: the presence of several introns in these genes, a circumstance that might increase the chances of occurrence of these events, and the presence of an efficient mechanism to keep low the mutation rate in the MHC region, thus preserving the sequences and thereby facilitating the exchange of segments.

4.4. Other important loci in mouse immunogenetics

The Tla

The Tla or TL complex is also located on chromosome 17 outside the MHC at about 1.5 cM from the H-2D region, and has been shown to control several cell-surface determinants, serologically defined. These antigens are only present on subpopulations of nucleated haematopoietic cells and are referred to as Qa 1 to Qa 8 and TL antigens. All of them are glycoproteins of molecular weights around 40 000, non-covalently associated to β2-microglobulin. Therefore it has been suggested that the Qa and TL antigens are biochemically and even functionally related to the K, D and L products of the H-2, although the TL antigens are not as similar as the Qa to these antigens. However, the Qa molecules do not seem to act as restrictor elements for cytotoxic T lymphocytes. No clear function has been assigned to these antigens, but in colony-forming cells the precursor cells of the megakaryocytes have been found to be Qa-2$^+$, while the precursors of macrophages, granulocytes, eosinophils and red cells are Qa-2$^-$, thus suggesting that they play a role in the differentiation of the bone marrow cells.

The T complex

The T complex is also located on chromosome 17 of the mouse, and contains variants with widely different characteristics involved in developmental processes. More than 10 mutants in this complex have been identified producing distinct embryological abnormalities. These range from the inability to form the blastocyst (homozygotes for the variant t^{12}), up to the development of a neural tube defect with other associated anomalies (t^{wl}/r^{wl}). The effects of these genes are implemented therefore very early in fetal development, within the first 10 days after fertilization.

A very interesting feature of this complex is that heterozygous males carrying the abnormal haplotype transmit it to their progeny in proportions that may approach 100% instead of the expected Mendelian proportions. It has been suggested therefore that the sperm carrying the abnormal haplotype is more effective in fertilization than those carrying the normal chromosome. As regards the serological aspects of this system, abnormal cell-surface antigens have been identified associated with the mutant T haplotypes, but only on the adult germ cells. These antigens seem to be glycoproteins of high molecular weight. A distinct antigen known as F9 may be one of these serological determinants since it is only found on sperm, early embryonic cells and in cultures of human embryonal carcinoma cells. The F9 antigen has a reciprocal expression with HLA antigens related to the stage of cell differentiation. There is also a structural similarity between the F9 antigen and the H-2 determinants. They are similar in molecular constitution and there is even the suggestion (though not yet proven) of expression of β2 microglobulin in the antigen.

4.5. *The minor histocompatibility system*

Besides the genes grouped in the MHC, there are also weak histocompatibility antigens under the control of a series of genes. More than 35 of these minor genes have so far been described together with some on the X and Y chromosomes.

There is also evidence that the immune response to some of these antigens may be coded for by genes within the H-2 system, and that the immunogenetic capacity of all the minor antigens is cumulatively equal to that of the MHS. There is nevertheless enormous variation in the immunogenicity of these minor antigens. The H-4B antigen for instance is slightly weaker than some of the H-2 antigens, while others like the H-9 are extremely weak.

The H-Y

To explain the graft rejection when a skin graft is transplanted from males to females of the same genetic constitution, the existence of a gene on the Y chromosome has been suggested, determining a specific male antigen. The function of this antigen is still debated, but it may be responsible for testicular development from the undifferentiated gonad. This antigen has also been studied in man, and is present in some individuals with testicular feminization, where the absence of testosterone receptors produces a female phenotype with normal male karyotype.

There are still problems with the H-Y antigen. For instance, although there is no doubt about its usual location on the Y chromosome, male mice have been observed with female chromosome constitutions (XX) but which are H-Y positive; in these it is suggested that another locus, Sxr, is responsible for the masculinization. To resolve the conflict with a location of H-Y on the Y chromosome, it has been suggested that the Sxr locus represents a translocation of a small piece of Y chromosome to one of the autosomes. However, definitions of the H-Y antigen are only operational, and it can be defined by a graft rejection, by killer cell action, or by serological methods.

The antigen THY1

This antigen is the most important marker of T lymphocytes in mice, although it is also found in other cells. Its locus seems to be on chromosome 9 and it produces a protein of molecular weight around 25 000.

The antigen LYM1

This is a serologically determined antigen whose product has similar properties to another one (the MLS) closely linked to it, and determined by mixed-lymphocyte culture. The identity of these two loci is not clear and they may be two different antigenic determinants expressed in a single molecule and the product of a single locus.

Ly antigens

These antigens are found in T and B lymphocytes, and are therefore named Lyt and Lyb respectively. These antigens are a group of products of various loci dispersed throughout the genome, whose only common function is their lymphocytotoxicity. For instance, the specificities Ly21 and Ly22; Ly31 and Ly32 are determined by one or two closely linked loci probably on the sixth chromosome of the mouse. Another group possibly located on the X chromosome has been detected and named LyX, predominantly expressed on T cells.

4.6. The human major histocompatibility system (HLA)

The equivalent in man to the H-2 system is located on the short arm of chromosome six and is known as HLA (Figure 4.2). Three types of genetic products are controlled by this region: two types of membrane proteins and some complement components. The polymorphic glycoproteins or surface antigens coded for by this group of genes include those classically known as transplant antigens or class I (HLA-A, HLA-B and HLA-C), and the immuno-associated or class II antigens coded for by genes at or around loci HLA-D and HLA-DR. Among the complement components known to be coded for by genes within the HLA are C4, C2 and factor B (BF) of the alternate pathway; these are known as class III products (Figure 4.2). The genes for receptors of some of the degradation products of C3 are also on chromosome 6.

The molecular structure and the general distribution of the antigens of the major histocompatibility complex are very similar in man and mouse, those of class I are associated with β2-microglobulin on the cell membrane, while the D/DR region is equivalent to the I region of the H-2. Hence, much of what has already been described applies to the HLA as well.

Serological versus lymphocytic determination

The determinants of the major histocompatibility complex have been studied basically by using two different techniques: using antibodies against the determinants (serological) and making use of the antigenicity of these determinants to stimulate the proliferative response of a set of cultured cells (lymphocytic). These different types of assays recognize different specificities, the HLA-A, B, C and DR being serologically defined, and the D specificities lymphocytically defined. Newer tests have helped in identifying new determinants. For instance, the primed lymphocyte test (PLT) identifies a set of determinants associated with the D region (see below).

The genetic map of the HLA system

It has been calculated that the chromosomal region covered by the HLA system has a length of more than 1.5 cM (some 3 000 kb), which is almost twice that of the H-2. Class I antigens in man seem to be located within a single region, in contrast to the mouse. The class II region (D region) is nearest to the centromere. The distance between the A locus and the centromere has been calculated to be between 6 and 14 cM and the locus of glyoxalase I (GLO) lies between the centromere and the HLA at about 4 cM from the latter. The HLA-D region of the MHC

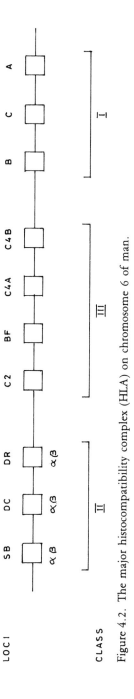

Figure 4.2. The major histocompatibility complex (HLA) on chromosome 6 of man.

is in many respects similar to the I region of the mouse. The initial studies of this region were restricted to the typing of the HLA-D determinants by mixed-lymphocyte culture. However, the development of serological methods for antigens within the same region brought about the identification of the DR series whose relationship with the former D antigens has not yet been clarified, but it is usually assumed that more than one antigen is involved in the mixed-lymphocyte culture stimulation and hence the D is more a region than a single locus.

Genetic, molecular and cellular analysis of the D region have led to the definition of various families of genes: the DR and DQ (including the DC, MB and DS of the old terminology), serologically defined, and the DP (formerly known as SB or PL-3) defined by the primed lymphocyte test. In the genetic map they seem to be located in the order DP–DQ–DR–B–C–A, from the centromere.

The molecular relationships of the human B-cell alloantigens are rather complex. There is a single α gene within the DR family, with various copies of the β gene. The DQ consists of two α genes, $DQ\alpha 1$ and $DQ\alpha 2$, and two β genes. The DP region has also two α and two β genes, $DP\alpha 1$, $\alpha 2$, $\beta 1$ and $\beta 2$. In addition to these genes, there is another α chain gene within the MHC, known as $DZ\alpha$, whose exact location and function is not yet known.

4.7. Molecular structure of the HLA genes

The general structure of the HLA products is similar to those of the H-2; the class I antigens are made up of a heavy chain and a β-2-microglobulin, and the class II composed of two molecules of similar molecular weight (Figure 4.3).

Recent studies of the complete nucleotide sequence of cDNA of a class I antigen showed the following characteristics.

1. A leader peptide encodes a stretch of 21 amino acids, 125 bp upstream of the first domain.

2. The first, second and third domains of the chain and the transmembrane segment are encoded by separate exons (2, 3, 4 and 5, respectively) separated by introns of varied lengths.

3. The exon 5 codes for: (*a*) a short hydrophilic segment (Glu-Pro-Ser-Ser), perhaps part of the third domain; (*b*) a stretch of 28 hydrophobic amino acids corresponding to the transmembrane segment; (*c*) a hydrophilic peptide (Met-Trp-Arg-Lys-Lys-Ser-Ser) which is the beginning of the cytoplasmic region and is considered to play a role in fastening the antigen to the cell membrane.

4. The cytoplasm is coded for by three exons, coding for seven, 11 and 14 amino acids, the first two separated by an intron of 438 nucleotides and a smaller one of 141 nucleotides between the second and third exons.

The DNA sequence of the heavy chain of the DR antigens shows 4 exons with the following characteristics:

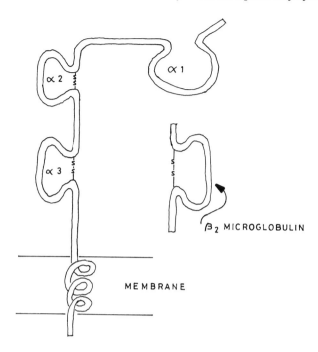

Figure 4.3. Diagrammatic representation of the molecular structure of class I histocompatibility antigens.

1. The first exon codes for the $\alpha 1$ domain, comprising amino acids 3–84.

2. The second codes for the $\alpha 2$ domain, amino acids 85–178, and bears a marked resemblance to the constant regions of the immunoglobulin.

3. The third encodes amino acids 179–288, consisting of a connecting peptide, the hydrophobic transmembrane segment and the hydrophilic intracytoplasmic carboxyl terminus, followed by a stop codon.

4. The fourth exon contains the remaining part of the 3′ untranslated region.

The cDNA analysis of the heavy chain of the DC1 antigen has shown it to be very similar to the DR, but the former has three amino acids more (232 and 229, respectively). Both the DR and DC1 molecules have one high mannose oligosaccharide moiety and one complex *N*-linked oligosaccharide moiety.

Assembly of the histocompatibility antigens

The assembly of the HLA antigens has been studied in some detail. As regards class I antigens, heavy chains and $\beta 2$-microglobulin are independently inserted into the membrane of the endoplasmic reticulum, and the assembly occurs within five minutes. It has already been mentioned that the attachment of

β2-microglobulin is a requirement for the intracellular transport of the HLA antigens. This conclusion is supported by the finding that Daudi cells, which do not synthesize β2-microglobulin, do not express heavy chain on the cell surface. From the endoplasmic reticulum, perhaps through transport vesicles, the antigens pass to the Golgi complex and finally to the cell membrane.

The DR antigens follow a similar pattern, being first inserted into the membrane of the endoplasmic reticulum and then transported via the Golgi complex to the cell surface. Three polypeptides are involved in this case: the α, β and γ chains. The assembly of the three chains takes place shortly after the synthesis but the γ chain is synthesized in excess and is therefore found free or combined with the α or the β chain. The molecular weight of the complex increases during its transport, probably because of the addition of sugars in the Golgi complex. This is followed by the detachment of the γ chain and the appearance of α and β chains on the cell surface.

4.8. Population studies

Although there is still much to be learned about the structure and genetic mechanisms of the HLA system, and the techniques to identify different loci are still improving, much reliable information has been obtained through the years regarding the population distribution of the HLA antigens (Figure 4.4). Table 4.1 lists the recognized antigens at each locus, according to the last workshop on histocompatibility. In clarification, the w prefix in some of the determinants means that they are not fully recognized as such by the histocompatibility workshop. Many factors are involved in this recognition. For instance, an antigen can be 'split' into others because they represent different antigenic specificities carried by the same molecule. This has been shown to be the case in many broad specificities as can be seen in Table 4.2. Cross-reactivity and the presence of private and public specificities (sometimes called short and long antigens) may complicate even further the definition of a given antigen.

Another interesting feature of the HLA polymorphism at the population level is the so-called linkage disequilibrium. This term means that some combinations of antigens tend to occur in the same haplotypes more frequently than would be expected by their gene frequencies. For instance, if the antigen HLA-A25 has a frequency of 0.04 (i.e. 4%) in a given population and the HLA-B13 has a frequency of 0.8 in the same population both antigens should be found together at a frequency of 0.032 (0.04×0.8) if the population under study has attained genetic equilibrium, and this rule holds even if the genes are linked. If in that population, however, the frequency is higher or lower then 0.032, the two antigens are said to be in linkage disequilibrium. The measure of linkage disequilibrium is called Δ and is the difference between the observed and expected values.

The pairs of antigens in linkage disequilibrium are not the same in every

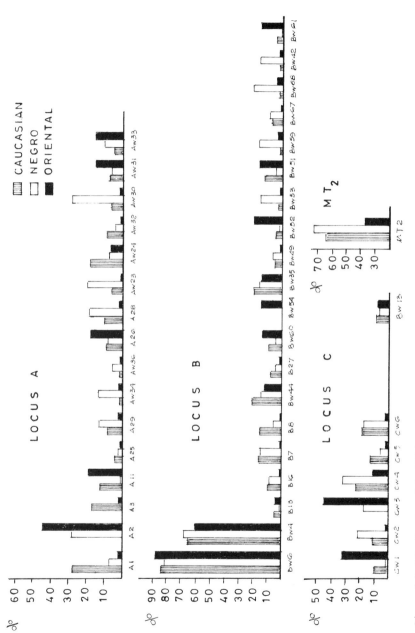

Figure 4.4. Distribution of the HLA antigens in Caucasians, Negroes and Orientals (data from the Histocompatibility Workshop 1980).

Human immunogenetics

Table 4.1. Nomenclature of the HLA alleles (1984).

A	B		C	D	DR	DQ	DP
A1	B5	Bw4	Cw1	Dw1	DR1	DQw1	DPw1
A2	B7	Bw6	Cw2	Dw2	DR2	DQw2	DPw2
A3	B8		Cw3	Dw3	DR3	DQw3	DPw3
A9	B12		Cw4	Dw4	DR4		DPw4
A10	B13		Cw5	Dw5	DR5		DPw5
A11	B14		Cw6	Dw6	DRw6		DPw6
Aw19	B15		Cw7	Dw7	DR7		
A23	B16		Cw8	Dw8	DRw8		
A24	B17			Dw9	DRw9		
A25	B18			Dw10	DRw10		
A26	B21			Dw11	DRw11		
A28	Bw22			Dw12	DRw12		
A29	B27			Dw13	DRw13		
A30	B35			Dw14	DRw14		
A31	B37			Dw15			
A32	B38			Dw16	DRw52		
Aw33	B39			Dw17	DRw53		
Aw34	B40			Dw18			
Aw36	Bw41			Dw19			
Aw43	Bw42						
Aw66	B44						
Aw68	B45						
Aw69	Bw46						
	Bw47						
	Bw48						
	B49						
	Bw50						
	B51						
	Bw52						
	Bw53						
	Bw54						
	Bw55						
	Bw56						
	Bw57						
	Bw58						
	Bw59						
	Bw60						
	Bw61						
	Bw62						
	Bw63						
	Bw64						
	Bw65						
	Bw66						
	Bw67						
	Bw70						
	Bw71						
	Bw72						
	Bw72						
	Bw73						

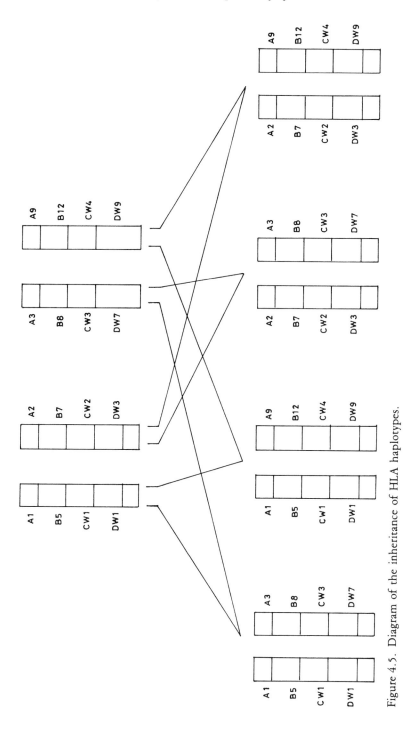

Figure 4.5. Diagram of the inheritance of HLA haplotypes.

Table 4.2. Splits of broad specificities according to the Histocompatibility Workshop, 1984.

Original broad specificities	Splits
A9	A23, A24
A10	A25, A26, Aw34, Aw66
Aw19	A29, A30, A31, A32, Aw33
A28	Aw68, Aw69
B5	B51, Bw52
B12	B44, B45
B14	Bw64, Bw65
B15	Bw62, Bw63
B16	B38, B39
B17	Bw57, Bw58
B21	B49, Bw50
Bw22	Bw54, Bw55, Bw56
B40	Bw60, Bw61
Bw70	Bw71, Bw72
DR5	DRw11, DRw12
DRw6	DRw13, DRw14
Dw6	Dw18, Dw19
Dw7	Dw11, Dw17

Inclusions of HLA-B specificities into Bw4 and Bw6.
Bw4: B5, B13, B17, B27, B37, B38 (16), B44 (12), Bw47, B49 (21), B51 (6), Bw52 (5), Bw53, Bw57 (17), Bw58 (17), Bw59, Bw63 (15).
BW6: B7, B8, B14, B18, Bw22, B35, B39 (16), B40, Bw41, Bw42, B45 (12), Bw46, Bw48, Bw50 (21), Bw54 (w22), Bw55 (w22), Bw56 (w22), Bw60 (40), BW61 (40), Bw62 (15), Bw64 (14), Bw57, Bw67, Bw71 (w70), Bw72 (w70), Bw73.

population, and this fact is taken into account when analysing the associations between HLA and disease.

At another genetic level, each parent provides each offspring with one of the two chromosomes 6 containing the HLA system. The combination of genes on each chromosome is called the haplotype. Of the four haplotypes available (two in the mother and two in the father) there are at fertilization four possible combinations, and the sibs have therefore a 25% probability of being HLA identical, 50% probability of having one haplotype in common, and 25% of being different in both haplotypes. Figure 4.5 shows the inheritance of the HLA haplotypes.

Bibliography

Amos, D. B. and Kostyu, D. D., HLA-A central immunological agency of man. *Adv. Hum. Genet.*, **10**: 137 (1980).
Auffray, C., Kuo, J., DeMars, R. and Strominger, J. L., A minimum of four human class

II α-chain genes are encoded in the HLA region of chromosome 6. *Nature*, **304**: 174 (1983).

Bach, F. H., The HLA class II genes and products: the HLA-D region. *Immunol. Today*, **6**(3): 89 (1985).

Barnstable, C. J., Jones, E. A. and Crumpton, M. J., Isolation, structure and genetics of HLA-A, -B, -C and -DRw (Ia) antigens. *Br. Med. Bull.*, **34**: 241 (1978).

Day, C. E. and Jones, P. P., The gene encoding the Ia antigen-associated invariant chain (Ii) is not linked to the H- 2 complex. *Nature*, **302**: 157 (1983).

Degos, L., Supertypic HLA-DR specificities. In *Histocompatibility Testing*. ULCA University Press, Los Angeles, pp. 570–571 (1980).

Delovitch, T. L. and Barber, B. H., Evidence for two homologous, but nonidentical, Ia molecules determined by the I-EC subregion. *J. Exp. Med.*, **150**: 100 (1979).

Gill III, T. J., Kunz, H. W., Schaid, D. J., Vandeberg, J. L. and Stolic, V., Orientation of loci in the major histocompatibility complex of the rat and its comparison to man and the mouse. *J. Immunogenet.*, **9**: 281 (1982).

Graff, R. J., Minor histocompatibility genes and their products. *Transplant. Proc.*, **10**: 701 (1978).

Ibstberg, L., Rask, L., Nillson, K. and Peterson, P. A., Independent expression of the two HL-A antigen polypeptide chains. *Eur. J. Immunol.*, **5**: 462 (1975).

Jonker, M. and Bainer, H., The major histocompatibility complex: a key to a better understanding of evolution. *Transplant. Proc.*, **12**: 575 (1980).

Karr, R. M., Kannapell, C. C., Stein, J. A., Gebel, H. M., Mann, D. L., Duquesnoy, R. J., Fuller, T. C., Rodey, G. E. and Schwartz, B. D., Molecular relationships of the B cell alloantigens, MT2, MB3, MT4 and DR5. *J. Immunol.*, **128**(4): 1809 (1982).

Korman, A. J., Auffray, C., Schamboeck, A. and Strominger, J. L., The amino acid sequence and gene organisation of the heavy chain of the HLA-DR antigen: homology to immunoglobulins. *Proc. Natl Acad. Sci. USA*, **79**: 6013 (1982).

Kvist, S., Wiman, K., Claesson, L., Peterson, P. A. and Dobberstein, B., Membrane insertion and oligomeric assembly of HLA-DR histocompatibility antigens. *Cell*, **29**: 61 (1982).

Lee, J. S., Trowsdale, J., Travers, P. J., Carey, J., Grosveld, F., Jenkins, J. and Bodmer, W. F., Sequence of an HLA-DR α-chain cDNA clone and intron-exon organisation of the corresponding gene. *Nature*, **299**: 750 (1982).

Malissen, M., Malissen, B. and Jordan, R., Exon/intron organisation and complete nucleotide sequence of an HLA gene. *Proc. Natl Acad. Sci. USA*, **79**: 893 (1982).

McDevitt, H., Mathis, D. and Monaco, J., I-region genes in mouse and man. *Tranplant. Proc.*, **15**: 50 (1983).

Ohta, T., Allelic and nonallelic homology of a supergene family. *Proc. Natl. Acad. Sci. USA*, **79**: 3251 (1982).

Olaisen, B., Teisberg, P., Jonassen, R., Thorsby, E. and Gedde-Dahl Jr, T., Gene order and gene distances in the HLA region studied by the haplotype method. *Ann. Hum. Genet.*, **47**: 285 (1983).

Owerbach, D., Lernmark, A., Rask, L., Peterson, P. A., Platz, P. and Svejgaard, A., Detection of HLA-D/DR-related DNA polymorphism in HLA-D homozygous typing cells. *Proc. Natl Acad. Sci. USA*, **80**: 3758 (1983).

Shaw, S., Kavathas, P., Pollack, M. S., Charmot, D. and Mawas, C., Family studies define a new histocompatibility locus, SB, between HLA-DR and GLO. *Nature*, **293**: 7451 (1981).

Simpson, E. and Gordon, R. D., Responsiveness to HY antigen Ir gene complementation and target cell specificity. *Immunological Rev.*, **35**: 59 (1977).

Snell, G. D., Recent advances in histocompatibility immunogenetics. *Adv. Genet.*, **20**: 291 (1979).

Sorrentino, R., Gorte, G., Calabi, F., Tanigaki, N. and Tosi, R., Microfingerprinting analysis of human Ia molecules favours a three loci model. *Mol. Immunol.*, **20**: 333 (1983).

Steinmetz, M., Minard, K., Horvath, S., McNicholas, J., Srelinger, J., Nake, C., Long, E., Mach, B. and Hood, L., A molecular map of the immune response region from the major histocompatibility complex of the mouse. *Nature*, **300**: 35 (1982).

Steinmetz, M., Winoto, A., Minard, K. and Hood, L., Clusters of genes encoding mouse transplantation antigens. *Cell*, **28**: 489 (1982).

Thorsby, E., Albrechtsen, D., Bergholtz, B. O., Hirschberg, H. and Solheim, B. G., Identification and significance of products of the HLA-D region. *Transplant. Proc.*, **10**: 313 (1978).

Watson, A. J., DeMars, R., Trowbridge, I. S. and Bach, F. H., Detection of a novel human class II HLA antigen. *Nature*, **304**: 358 (1983).

Winoto, A., Steinmetz, M. and Hood, L., Genetic mapping in the major histocompatibility complex by restriction enzyme site polymorphisms: most mouse class I antigens map to the Tla complex. *Proc. Natl Acad. Sci. USA*, **80**: 3425 (1983).

Chapter 5. The genetic control of immune responses

So far, in examining various types of genetic control over the immune system, we have seen that there is strong genetic determination of features of the MHC, and some genetic influence on the circulating levels of the immunoglobulins, and on the synthesis and control of some other mediators of the immune response. At another level, the genetic defects in some of the immune proteins have obvious repercussions in the immune competence of the individual. However, when referring to the genetic control of the immune response, it is not genetic control of the total immunity that is meant, but of the capacity to respond to a single antigen of restricted heterogeneity and specificity.

The first experiments showing a genetic control of this kind were performed using inbred mice and guinea-pigs immunized with simple synthetic polypeptides like poly-L-lysine (PLL) and the co-polymer of L-glutamic acid and L-lysine (GL). These experiments showed that some animals were capable of mounting an immune response to these antigens as measured by delayed hypersensitivity and the production of specific antibodies, while others did not. Responsiveness and nonresponsiveness were also shown to be inherited in a clear Mendelian fashion, controlled by autosomal dominant genes, now known as *Ir* genes. Soon after, it was found that these genes mapped within the H-2 system of the mouse.

For some years, the nature of the *Ir* gene-products was unknown, and the *Ir* genes themselves were believed to lie within the major histocompatibility complex but as entities distinct from the other determinants coded for by this complex, and perhaps involved in the synthesis of the T-cell receptors. Moreover, the description of a set of determinants capable of inducing the formation of antibodies in mice immunized with cells from strains only differing in their *Ir* genes, the immuno-associated or *Ia* genes, complicated the problem even more, for they also mapped within the MHC and were very close to the putative position of the *Ir* genes.

As already mentioned, the *Ir* genes are known today to code for the Ia determinants, and the clue to understanding the genetic control of immune responses and hence the *Ir* genes is to be found in the restriction mechanism of the major histocompatibility complex.

T lymphocytes, when presented with an antigen in the right manner, react in one of two ways: through the generation of T-cytotoxic lymphocytes (T_c) or through amplification (T_h) or suppression (T_s) of the effects of other T or B cells. In general, T lymphocytes only recognize the antigen and respond to it when it is presented on the surface of an 'antigen-presenting cell'. This 'antigen-presenting cell' may vary according to the type of T lymphocyte involved. Thus, in the generation of cytotoxic responses, lymphocytes and perhaps macrophages are the cells involved in presenting the antigen to the T_c cells, while in the other types of T response the presenting cell seems to be the macrophage and perhaps the dendritic cells.

5.1. Interaction between T cells in the cytotoxic response

So far, in studies on cytotoxic responses to viral and minor histocompatibility antigens as well as those involved in cell-mediated lympholysis against allo-antigens, T_c lymphocytes require T_h lymphocytes for the induction of the response. The process of generating T_c cells takes place in two steps. First, the antigen is presented to T cells, perhaps by the macrophage, and precursor T_c cells recognize it in the context of class I antigens. As a result of this first antigenic contact, the T_c precursors become 'conditioned' and express a new receptor on their surface, specific for a factor known as T-cell growth factor (TCGF) or interleukin-2 (IL-2). The IL-2 is released by T_h lymphocytes (Lyt-1^+, 23^- in mice and $T4^+$ in man). The second step is the binding of IL-2 to the new receptors of the T_c precursors. At the same time, T_h cells need to be conditioned by a similar process before they release the IL-2. In this case, T_h lymphocytes (Lyt-1^+, 23^-) recognize the antigen on the surface of a macrophage in the context of a class II antigen, and the macrophage releases another mediator (interleukin-1 or IL-1) that binds a receptor on the T_h surface. It is clear, therefore, that the T_h lymphocytes are restricted here by class II antigens, while the T_c cells (Lyt-1^-, 23^+) themselves are restricted by class I antigens. The role of the Lyt antigens in this interaction is far from clear. It has been suggested that the Lyt-2 antigens may be involved in the stabilization of the initial contact between the antigen and the cellular receptor. However, it is a general rule only that T_h cells are restricted by class II products, for exceptions are known. Furthermore, cytotoxic reactions have been blocked by the administration of anti-Lyt-2, which taken jointly with some other data indicate that the anti-Lyt-2 antibodies are inhibiting the antigen-recognition process. Hence, these antigens may play a very important role in the T-cell responses, perhaps in association with the MHC molecules.

Other types of cytotoxic responses

Although all the known cytotoxic responses to foreign antigens are, as seen above, restricted by class I antigens, it seems that class II molecules may also be involved.

This occurs in particular in the cytotoxic responses to alloantigens of the MHC — when the MHC molecules are being considered as a foreign antigen — although here again class I antigens may also be involved.

5.2. B-cell responses

For B cells to be activated, binding to the antigen is necessary, plus a second signal, usually given by a T_h lymphocyte. However, the T_h lymphocytes require the presentation of the antigen in a processed form by an adequate antigen-presenting cell, and in the context of the MHC determinants (class II). In this case the type of antigen-presenting cell is likely to be a macrophage or a dendritic cell, but other cell types, especially B cells, can also process the antigen and present it in the context of class II molecules. It has nevertheless been established that whatever the antigen-presenting cell is, it has to process the antigen before presenting it to the T_h lymphocytes. This involves taking up the antigen, sequestering it in intracellular compartments and re-expressing it on the cell surface. There is considerable evidence that soluble protein antigens are not recognized by the T_h lymphocyte in their native form. Recent evidence, however, shows that fragmentation of the antigen may be enough at least for some systems so that they may be recognized in association with class II molecules.

Expression density of class II products

It is clear that while class II antigens are present on all B cells, the density of expression of these antigens is rather heterogeneous, and it seems that this quantitative expression may be critical in B-cell activation. In fact, it has been shown that B cells with high levels of class II expression are more easily activated by T_h cells.

T–B interaction

Little is known about the molecular relationship that must take place during the T_h–B cell interaction. Certainly, part of this lack of knowledge seems to be due to the fact that there are various types of B cells with different behaviours when confronting the T cell. At least two such subpopulations have been identified by their expression of the Lyb-5 determinant: and it seems that only those Lyb-5$^-$ when interacting with the T_h lymphocyte are restricted by the MHC (Class II) antigens; the activation of the Lyb-5$^+$ B cells occurs without direct interaction between T_h and B cells.

5.3. Nonresponsiveness

It has been pointed out that class I molecules are necessary for the recognition of foreign antigens (discrimination between self and non-self) while the class II determinants are used by the immune system to recognize its own cells during the process of cell co-operation. The Ia antigens in mice (Ia-like in man), coded for by the *Ir* genes, are the same as the class II molecules, and hence the responsiveness and nonresponsiveness originally ascribed to separate Ir entities may well be understood as a defect in the process of recognition of class II determinants.

'Ir genes'

There is now evidence that what were interpreted as the effects of *Ir* genes are instead due to failure of the MHC restriction, and it is very unlikely that *Ir* genes exist as separate entities.

If in given animal strains the response and nonresponse to a single antigen behave in a Mendelian form, and map, say, to the I-A region of the H-2, then if this responsiveness were due to the expression of the I-A antigen on the lymphocyte surface, one could induce nonresponsiveness by adding anti-I-A antibodies to the responder's lymphocytes, and not by adding any other anti-H-2 antibodies. This is in fact what some investigators have observed by means of monoclonal antibodies of very high specificity, arguing in favour of the restriction mechanism as the underlying basis for the genetic control of immune responses. From these experiments three important points emerge:

1. In responder strains some antigens are recognized by the I-A molecules and others by the I-E molecules. Examples of I-A restricted are the poly(Glu^{40} Ala^{60}) or GA and the response to lactate dehydrogenase B. The responses to GLPhe and GLT are restricted by I-E molecules.
2. This choice of Ia determinant is invariable for each antigen in all different responder haplotypes.
3. Blocking the correct restriction molecule to a given antigen does not induce a switch to another one (i.e., in the response to GA, blocking the I-A molecule will not induce a response through the I-E molecule).

Hence, if the choice of restriction molecule is invariable for any given antigen and cannot be changed during an immune response, one may wonder how and when the selection was done. No clear explanation is available for these questions so far, but two possibilities have been put forward:

1. In early T-cell ontogeny the individual has both A and E restricting cells and eliminates one of them during development.
2. The selection, perhaps genetic, is done early and the individual only develops either A or E restricting cells.

The nonresponsiveness at the functional level

Finally, some mechanism is necessary to explain why the I-A or I-E molecules, although present, do not function properly in nonresponder individuals. Again, here experimental demonstrations are not yet available, and hence various hypotheses have been suggested.

1. The complex antigen-Ia molecule is not recognized by the T cell because of a failure at the level of the antigen-presenting cells.
2. There is simultaneous stimulation of suppressor T cells by some combinations of antigen and Ia molecules.
3. There is a lack in some individuals of specific subsets of T_h cells to recognize specific combinations of antigen-Ia molecules.

Evidence is available regarding the existence of suppressor T cells (T_s) in some types of nonresponsiveness and they are thought to be produced by the action of immune-suppression or *Is* genes, with the same connotations as the MHC restriction of the *Ir* genes.

5.4. The T-cell receptor

The fact that T cells need to recognize two structures (the foreign antigen and the MHC molecule) for their subsequent activation has posed some problems in speculations on the structure of the T-cell receptor, particularly whether there are two separate receptors, or a single receptor for the combination of antigen and MHC determinant. The latter is called the 'altered self' receptor, which is favoured by many, since formal proof for one or the other is still lacking.

More recently, new models have been suggested. One of them envisages a receptor made up of three separate structures: one for the MHC class, one for the polymorphic part of the histocompatibility antigen, and a third for the foreign antigen. The other model gives even more stress to the role of the cell-surface proteins of the lymphocyte: the human T cells with T8 on their surface (cytotoxic and supressor functions) would interact with class I antigens through the T8 and T3 structure, composed of a clonally unique glycoprotein subunit (Ti) in association with the T3 molecule. The T4 lymphocytes (inducer cells) would interact with class II antigens by the T4 and the same T3 structure. In fact, recent serological and molecular genetic analysis of T-cell clones have shown that the receptor of the T cell is made up of two glycosylated, disulphide-linked polypeptide chains (Tiα and Tiβ), both spanning the cell membrane, associated with the T3 complex consisting of a 25-kDa chain and two subunits with molecular weights of 20 kDa. The cloning of the genes encoding the two chains from mouse and human DNA revealed that α and β chains have variable and constant regions; the Tiβ consists of two tandemly arranged sets of segments called D_{B1}-J_{B1}-C_{B1} and D_{B2}-J_{B2}-C_{B2}. The two constant regions differ only in six amino acids in the translated regions. There is also a V gene pool located 5′ at an unknown distance from the D_1 segment. Similar analysis of the Tiα indicates that these molecules are also homologous in structure to the immunoglobulin genes, and it is therefore likely that both Tiα and Tiβ subunits interact to form a single combining site

for the antigen and the MHC molecule. The relationship between immunoglobulins and the T-cell receptor is supported by the fact that the $Ti\beta$ chain
genes and the $\varkappa$ light-chain genes are closely linked in the mouse (chromosome
6) although not in humans (chromosomes 7 and 2, respectively), and also by the
fact that the $Ti\alpha$ genes are linked in the mouse to the purine nucleoside
phosphorylase gene (chromosome 14) whose deficiency is associated with a T-cell
immune deficiency in man (see Chapter 8).

Bibliography

Acuto, D. and Reinherz, E. L., The human T-cell receptor. *New Engl. J. Med.*, **312**(17):
    1100 (1985).
Benacerraf, B., Role of MHC gene products in immune regulation. *Science*, **212**: 1229
    (1981).
Benacerraf, B. and McDevitt, H. O., Histocompatibility-linked immune response genes.
    Science, **175**: 273 (1972).
Davis, B. K., Shonnard, J. W., Cramer, D. V. and Lobel, S. A., The immune response
    to poly(Glu^{52}Lys^{33}Tyr^{15}) in inbred and wild rats. *Transplant Proc.*, **11**: 1593 (1979).
Dembic, Z., Bannwarth, W., Taylor, B. A. and Steinmetz, M., The gene encoding the
    T-cell receptor α-chain maps close to the Np-2 locus on mouse chromosome 14.
    Nature, **314**: 271 (1985).
Eardley, D. D., Shen, F. W., Cantor, H. and Gershon, R. R., Genetic control of immuno-
    regulatory circuits. *J. Exp. Med.*, **150**: 100 (1979).
McMichael, A. J., Ting, A., Zweerink, B. J. and Askonas, B. A., HLA restriction of cell
    mediated lysis of influenza virus infected human cells. *Nature*, **270**: 524 (1977).
Mozes, E., Expression of immune response (Ir) genes in T and B cells. *Immunogenetics*,
    2: 397 (1975).
Munro, A. J. and Taussig, M. J., Two genes in the major histocompatibility complex con-
    trol immune response. *Nature*, **265**: 103 (1975).
Nagy, Z. A., Baxevanis, C. N., Ishii, N. and Klein, J., Ia antigens as restriction molecules
    in Ir-gene controlled T-cell proliferation. *Immunological Rev.*, **60**: 59 (1981).
Reinherz, E. L., Meuser, S. C. and Schlossman, S. F., The human T cell receptor: analysis
    with cytotoxic T cell clones. *Immunological Rev.*, **74**: 83 (1983).
Rock, K. L., The role of Ia molecules in the activation of T lymphocytes. *J. Immunol.*,
    129(4): 1360 (1982).
Talmage, D. W., Recognition and memory in the cells of the immune system. *Am. Sci.*,
    67: 173 (1979).
Taussig, M. J., Mozes, E. and Issac, R., Antigen specific thymic cell factors in the genetic
    control of the immune response to poly-(tyrosil glutamyl)-poly-D,L-alanyl-poly-lysil.
    J. Exp. Med., **140**: 301 (1974).
Uhr, J. W., Capra, D., Vitetta, E. S. and Cook, R. G., Organisation of the immune
    response genes. *Science*, **206**: 292 (1979).

Chapter 6. The genetics of the complement system

The complex complement system consists of a series of interacting plasma proteins which forms the principal effector arm of the antibody-mediated immune reactions. The basic chemistry of the system is well known and, more recently, the study of its genetic control has enormously expanded.

Basically there are three features of the system where genetic determination or control has been established:

1. The genetic polymorphisms that have been described for various individual components, of which C3 is the best studied.

2. The genetic contribution to the control of the levels of some of these components that started with the Ss protein in the mouse and that has been extended to its human equivalent.

3. The deficiencies of isolated components that have been shown to be inherited in a Mendelian fashion.

This chapter will discuss the genetic mechanisms involved in this variation.

6.1. The third component (C3)

Structure of the C3 molecule

C3 is synthesized as a single peptide, proC3, and then cleaved into two chains, a small, β, and a large, α, that are bound together by disulphide bridges to give the final C3 molecule of molecular weight around 198 000. The sequential breakdown of the C3 molecule produces a series of smaller molecules, preserving the double-chain structure in C3b, C3bi and C3c, and becoming a single α chain in C3d,g; C3d and C3j. For instance, C3c consists of one fragment from the β chain (MW 65–75 000) and two from the α chain (MW 4 000 and 22 000), the smaller being the amino-terminal end of the α chain.

The *C3* gene

Although there are clear differences between the nucleotide sequences of mouse and human C3 genes, the underlying homology allows the use of mouse cDNA as probes of their human equivalent. One celomic cDNA human clone containing the sequence of part of the α chain has already been isolated.

Structural polymorphism of C3

The genetic variants of C3 are detectable by high-voltage electrophoresis in agarose, followed by protein staining with amido-black. The use of Ca^{++} aids the identification of the bands, for it retards the migration of C3 relative to the other β-globulins. Using these standard techniques, over 20 variants of C3 have been identified, the commonest being those designated as S and F. The other variants have been named according to their migration distance relative to that between C3S and a rare variant, C3F1.0, being expressed as a decimal of the latter. The inheritance of the C3 variants has been confirmed to be autosomal co-dominant. Figure 6.1 shows some of these variants and their relative mobility.

The changes in the structure of C3 that are responsible for its variation are not known. It seems, nevertheless, that the differences between C3S and C3F are within the C3c portion of the molecule, and this is supported by the fact that the C3a derived from both the C3S and C3F has the same electrophoretic mobility. Moreover, using two-dimensional electrophoresis it has been observed that the common variants have charge differences located on the β chain.

So far there is no explanation for the existence of this polymorphism. Indeed, neither the haemolytic efficiency nor the serum concentration differ between individuals with different phenotypes. The serum concentrations are also similar for the different phenotypes during pregnancy and in the newborn period, as well

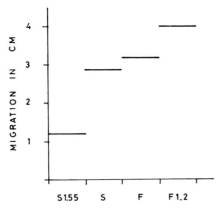

Figure 6.1. Position of the common S and F variants of C3 relative to the slower S1.55 and the faster F1.2.

as in normal adults of both sexes. In one study, however, the ability of C3S to induce the formation of rosettes between mononuclear cells and erythrocytes was found to be significantly less than that of the C3F serum. Similarly, the frequency of C3F was higher in mothers of ABO-incompatible babies with high antibody titres than in those with low antibody titres.

Foetal synthesis of C3 has been shown by discrepancies in the C3 types in maternal and cord sera. The liver was identified as the main site of synthesis of this complement component when an individual changed his type to that of the donor after undergoing liver transplantation. However, C3 is also synthesized outside the liver by other tissues and cells, among them the macrophages, monocytes, lymphoid cells, and synovial tissue in patients with rheumatoid arthritis but not in other types of joint disease. An interesting finding is that the C3 produced by the monocytes is functionally inactive for as yet unknown, but perhaps molecular, reasons.

The human C3 locus has been assigned, by somatic cell hybridization, to chromosome 19, closely linked to the loci for the Lewis blood group and for myotonic dystrophy. The most likely sequence of these and other linked genes seems to be Lewis–C3–myotonic dystrophy–secretor–peptidase D–Lutheran blood group.

Extensive population studies have been made on this polymorphism (Figure 6.2). In general, most is known about European populations. From Germany alone there are 12 different studies covering more than 10 000 individuals. These samples show a range of frequency for the *C3F* gene between 19 and 22%. Scandinavian populations are nearly as well represented, for there are eight studies covering over 6 000 individuals, and in almost all of them the gene frequency for C3F varies between 17 and 23%. Icelandic, English, Belgian, Dutch and Yugoslav samples show similar levels. Spain shows a slightly higher frequency but also within the European range (20–23%), as do Bulgarians and Georgians. As a whole, the frequency distribution of these genes is very homogeneous in Europe, and the frequencies persist in overseas peoples of European origin (North America and Australia). Of the two peoples in Europe who differ from other European populations in frequencies of other genetic markers, Basques show no difference for C3, but Lapps do differ in having a very low frequency of the *F* gene (2–7%). In India, two reports show the frequency of the *F* gene to be low as well (2.5%–10%), but there are some intra-population differences, for urban samples show a higher *C3F* gene frequency than their rural counterparts. A similar feature in Europe with Lapps and USSR Maris suggests that there may be a selective effect of urbanization on this polymorphism.

The other interesting features of the C3 polymorphism at the world level is that both Iran and Iraq show *C3F* gene frequencies similar to the European range, but in Afghanistan the frequency starts to decline, starting a gradient that persists into the Indian subcontinent. In Africa the *C3F* gene frequency in the few peoples studied also shows low levels of 2–6%.

The rare variants of this polymorphism also are of interest in their world

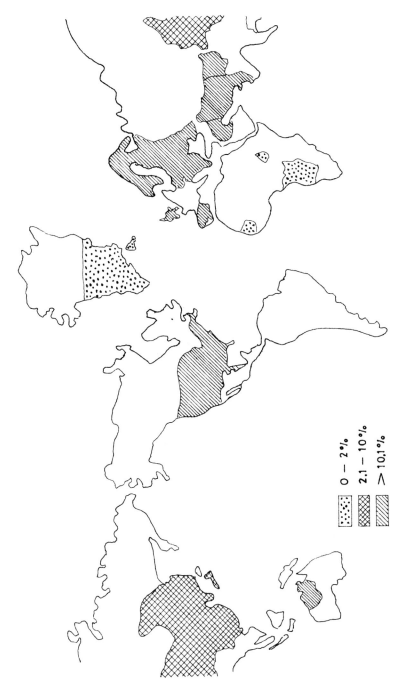

Figure 6.2. Gene frequency of C3F in various world populations.

distribution. The commonest variant seems to be the C3S0.4, with a frequency of about 1 in 200 Europeans. All the others show frequencies lower than 1 in 1000 individuals. Apart from the C3F0.7 and C3F0.8 that seem to be peculiar to Japan, no other variant is characteristic of a single population.

Again at the DNA level, restriction length polymorphisms have been described for C3, which means that there are differences in intron—exon sequences between individuals, although they all code identical proteins.

The mouse C3

Contrary to the observations in man, the C3 locus in mouse is linked to the MHC on chromosome 17. It has been observed by recombinant DNA technology that a single copy of the *C3* gene is contained in the mouse genome, which is important to the understanding of the mechanisms involved in the synthesis of the protein by specific tissues and in those responsible for the changes in levels observed in certain pathological conditions. The C3 gene in the mouse has been isolated, but its precise map has not been described yet. According to preliminary data, the gene is 1.2 kb long, and contains a 'TATA-box' (a typical sequence in promoter regions of eukaryotic genes), a leader peptide and three exons.

6.2. Factor B (BF)

Structure of the molecule and gene

Factor B is a single glycoprotein of molecular weight 90 000 which can be cleaved into two fragments: the Bb (MW 60 000) and the Ba (MW 30 000). Recently a membrane form of factor B has been described, but so far it is not known whether it is a membrane protein or the circulating form absorbed on to the cell surface.

The human cDNA clones have now been isolated and the structure of the BF gene determined. It spans 15 kb of genomic DNA, present only once in the human genome, and no pseudogenes have been identified. No restriction length polymorphism has been described for this gene.

Structural polymorphism of Factor B

The different phenotypes of Factor B are detected by electrophoresis in agarose followed by immunofixation with antiserum specific to Factor B. In this way two main bands are observed in the heterozygote, but, depending upon small variations in the technique, two or three more bands of lower intensity can be seen. As with the C3 system, the BF types are classified as F and S. Two less common variants observed are designated as F1 (faster than F) and S0.7 (slower than S) (Figure 6.3). These types are also inherited as autosomal co-dominant traits.

The structural changes in the BF molecule responsible for the genetic variants are not known, but it seems clear that, of the two major cleavage products, the

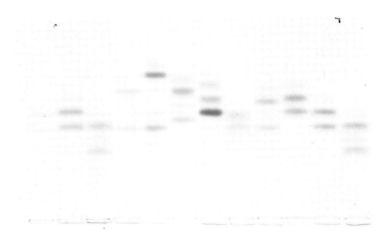

Figure 6.3. Electrophoretic variants of the BF system: factor B phenotypes are shown after high voltage agarose gel electrophoresis and anti-BF immunofixation common S (lanes 2, 3, 4, 6), F (lane 9) and SF (lanes 1, 5) alleles as well as "rare" variants F_1 (lane 7) and $S_{0.7}$ (lanes 8, 10–13) are shown.
(Photograph courtesy of G. Keyeux, Universidad Javeriana, Bogota, Colombia)

F and S variants are located on the Ba fragment, while the F1 and S0.7 are located on the Bb fragment.

So far no functional difference has been observed for the different phenotypes. During the course of our own studies of diabetics, we have found that individuals of the F type have significantly lower levels of circulating C3 than individuals of the S type, while the heterozygotes have intermediate levels. The importance of this finding is however not clear. More recently, the allotype BFF was found to be strongly associated with cytotoxic antibody production in multiparous women.

Population variation of the BF polymorphism has also been shown, although it is not as well documented as that of C3. Table 6.1 shows the gene frequencies of the populations so far studied, and it can be seen that the highest F gene frequencies are among peoples of Negro origin (up to 50%). So far only one sample from the Far East has been studied, showing the lowest F gene frequency of those described (11%). The few European studies do not permit a detailed discussion of the distribution of these alleles, but all of them seem to fall within the range of 15–25% for the F gene, and the one sample of Persians, as for C3, shows similarity to the European values. The only study available for Indian populations, although too restricted to be indicative of the entire Indian subcontinent, shows a pattern for BF different from that of C3. The frequency of the F allele is higher in Indian than in European populations, but not as high as in Negroid peoples. The studies so far described are thus still too fragmentary for full description of gene frequency distribution, but it is clear that the BF system is also useful in the study of populations. Whether this polymorphism shows similar frequency gradients to those seen for C3 remains to be investigated, but it may

Table 6.1. Distribution of *BF* alleles in various populations.

Population	N	*S*	*F*	S_1	F_1	$F_{1.6}$	Source
Swiss	654	0.805	0.176	0.009	0.010	—	Scherz *et al.* (1977)
Italian	62	0.718	0.250	0.024	0.008	—	Scherz *et al.* (1977)
West German	1245	0.808	0.1743	0.009	0.008	0.004	Mauff *et al.* (1975)
German	82	0.826	0.1492	0.012	0.012	—	Rittner *et al.* (1975)
Negroid	127	0.437	0.512	—	0.051	—	Alper *et al.* (1972)
Oriental	86	0.890	0.110	0.013	—	—	Alper *et al.* (1972)
Caucasian	158	0.709	0.278	—	—	—	Alper *et al.* (1972)
French	200	0.78	0.215	0.012	0.080	—	Marcelli *et al.* (1972)
Norwegian	172	0.814	0.174	0.006	0.006	—	Olafsen *et al.* (1975)
South African	224	0.435	0.513	0.018	0.029	—	Mauff *et al.* (1976)
South African	90	0.644	0.322	0.033	—	—	Mauff *et al.* (1976)
Negroids	944	0.282	0.655	—	—	—	Mauff *et al.* (1976)
Persian	99	0.727	0.257	0.015	—	—	Bernal *et al.* (1979)
Hindi	99	0.606	0.394	—	—	—	Bernal *et al.* (1979)
English	73	0.732	0.256	—	0.012	—	Bernal *et al.* (1979)

BF Alleles

be that different selective factors have been engaged in maintaining the two polymorphisms.

Linkage of BF and the HLA system was first demonstrated in 1974 in a study of 12 two-generation families segregating for BF, confirmed by further studies. One study where five HLA-BF recombinants were found among 82 informative meiotic divisions suggested that the BF locus is situated between the HLA-D and -B loci on chromosome 6, although its definitive position is not yet clear. There are, however, more than 400 informative meioses available with around 10 recombinants for HLA-B-BF. It gives an overall recombination frequency of more than twice that expected for HLA-B and HLA-D, and hence it is difficult to place the BF locus between the B and D loci, lending support to its location outside the D region.

These studies used the observation of recombinational events within families, which are rare because the loci are tightly linked. A method recently reported makes use of the linkage disequilibrium already mentioned as a peculiar characteristic of the HLA system, arguing as follows. A haplotype in linkage disequilibrium is that which occurs more often than expected from the frequency of its constituent alleles, and hence most of the alleles of low frequency will usually be found in disequilibrium in the same haplotype. Other haplotypes involving this allele will most probably be due to recombination. This nice argument led to the suggestion that the complement components lie between B and DR, in the order BF, C4B, C4A, C2 from the centromere (Chapter 4).

Of particular interest is the existence of a marked linkage disequilibrium between some of the *BF* alleles and the A and B loci of the HLA. The most significant is that between the *F1* variant and the *HLA-B18*. Others are between *BFS* and *HLA-B8* and between *BFS0.7* and *HLA-B12*, *B27*, *B13*, *B14* and *Bw21*. The split of *B21* into two sub-specificities (*B49* and *Bw50*) has shown that the linkage disequilibrium is between *BFS0.7* and *HLA Bw50*.

6.3. The fourth component (C4)

Molecular structure

The human C4 molecule is synthesized as a single chain (pro-C4) by the liver, monocytes and macrophages, and then split into three polypeptides α (MW 95 000), β (MW 75 000) and γ (MW 30 000) which are covalently linked. It has been observed that there are various different forms of C4 in plasma. After the synthesis, the pro-C4 undergoes intracellular proteolytic cleavage yielding the secreted form ($C4^s$) of the molecule, which accounts for around 10% of the total plasma C4. The predominant form in plasma ($C4^P$) has an α chain slightly smaller than that of the $C4^s$. During the activation of the complement system this native form is broken into C4a (MW 9 000) and C4b, the former being part of the amino terminal end of the α chain.

There are two concepts of the genetics of human C4. One proposes the existence of two closely linked loci, not allelic to each other, and the other is not committed to the number of loci and their genetic interrelationship. The two structural linked loci so far identified are within the *MHC* and are known as C4A (previously called F) and C4B (previously called S). The products of these respective loci absorbed on to the membrane of the erythrocyte correspond to what were previously known as the Chido and Rodgers blood groups. The antisera against these blood groups apparently detect antigenic determinants in the α chain of C4.

The genetic polymorphism of C4 has been located in the α chain of the molecule; in fact, α chains of the C4A seem to be larger than those of the C4B but less functional. Recently, five different forms of the β chain were observed in members of 32 German families, indicating that there is also a structural polymorphism at this level of the molecule.

The nomenclature of the C4 bands observed in desialized plasma is rather complex. Figure 6.4 shows some of the variants. Each allotype pattern usually consists of anodal and cathodal bands, the latter usually being minor. These allotypes are numbered from A1 to A6 and from B1 to B7; the alleles are distinguished from the allotypes by an asterisk after the letter of the locus (e.g. *C4B**). The non-expressed alleles are referred to as *QO*, for instance *C4A*QO*.

Another interesting feature of the genetics of C4 is the genetic control of the circulating levels of the protein, observed in the mouse model and also in man. It has been observed in this respect that the different phenotypes in man correspond to different circulating levels, but the genetic mechanism for this is far from clear and further investigation with the recently developed methods of C4 typing is needed.

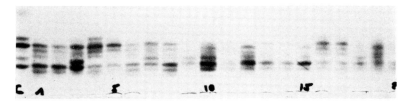

Figure 6.4. Electrophoretic and immunofixation of C4. C4 phenotypes are shown after high voltage agarose gel electrophoresis and anti-C4 immunofixation products from the C4A locus migrate faster towards the anode than the C4B locus products, and both main bands can be clearly distinguished from the several minor bands.
C: control A3,3 B1,1 serum.
(Photograph courtesy of G Keyeux, Universidad Javeriana, Bogota, Colombia)

As for Factor B, linkage disequilibrium has been observed between C4 and the HLA system.

6.4. Other components

The second component (C2)

The second component of complement is a single peptide of molecular weight around 100 000 which is split into two fragments, C2a (MW 70 000) and C2b (MW 30 000) when activation of the complement occurs.

Structural polymorphism of C2 has also been described linked to the HLA system. By isoelectric focusing two alleles, $C2^1$ and $C2^2$ are normally found in populations, the $C2^1$ with a frequency around 95–97%. A third rarer allele, $C2^3$, is found with a very low frequency (1%) in Europeans.

The sixth component (C6)

The human C6 consists of a single polypeptide of molecular weight around 105 000 and a carbohydrate content between 4 and 10%. Typing of human C6 can be performed either by agarose electrophoresis followed by immunofixation, or by isoelectric focusing, the latter giving rather better results. With both techniques an extensive polymorphism has been observed, with at least six bands of different intensity. The phenotypes have been named A and B (for acidic and basic), the heterozygotes giving a pattern of superimposition of those of the homozygous A and B. The inheritance of these C6 types has been shown to be autosomal co-dominant.

As with other complement components, differences between maternal and cord serum C6 types indicate that it does not cross the placenta and that the fetus synthesizes its own C6.

Gene frequencies for a few populations are available showing that there are small differences between the major ethnic groups, the $C6^*A$ being the commonest type (56–61%) in most populations. Rare variants have been observed with frequencies up to 6%, which are inherited also as autosomal co-dominants, their genes behaving as alleles of the common variants.

The C6 locus is not closely linked to the HLA system, although there is a report of a small positive lod score for C6-HLA linkage in male meiosis and another report of linkage, but at a map distance of more than 15 cM from the HLA-B.

The seventh component (C7)

Human C7 is a single polypeptide of molecular weight 92 000 with a carbohydrate content of 6%, and homology between this protein and C6 has been suggested based on amino acid composition, size and chain structure. More recent work taking into account the chemical properties of both molecules as well as sequence analysis of the amino end do not confirm the presumed homology. Moreover, C7 was shown in this study to be more similar to Factor B than to C6. The apparent similarity in the structural polymorphism of both components suggested also that their loci were linked.

Allotypes of C7 have been described, with the commonest variant being present in about 99% of people. Although its locus is not yet assigned, the possible linkage to C6, and the loose association of C6 to the HLA system, place it provisionally around 15 cM from the major histocompatibility system on the 6th chromosome.

The eighth component (C8)

Human C8 has a molecular weight of 151 000 and is composed of three non-identical molecules; α (MW 64 000), β (MW 64 000) and γ (MW 22 000). This molecule occurs as a dimer α-γ covalently linked, which is non-covalently associated with the β chain. It is not clear whether the three chains are synthesized as a single peptide and broken down into the subunits (like C4 and C3).

Structural polymorphism for this complement component has also been described but does not seem to be linked to the HLA system.

6.5. The genetic control of the complement levels

Besides the genetic control of most of the complement components at the structural level, there are indications that genes may also control the circulating levels of some of them. The first indication of this type of genetic control came from studies in mice where the Ss protein, later identified as mouse C4, was found to be quantitatively controlled by a gene within the major histocompatibility complex. The question was then whether similar genes existed for human complement. Low concentrations, presumably due to heterozygosity for a deficiency gene, have been reported for C4, C2, BF and C3. For C4 and C2 the frequency of these low concentrations in a population is relatively high, particularly among HLA-B18 and HLA-DW2 individuals where about 9% are heterozygous for the putative deficiency gene.

In the course of our own studies we have found a high incidence of low C4 levels in patients with spinal muscular atrophy and their relatives. In total, seven out of 34 patients and 22 of their relatives studied showed levels presumably due to heterozygosity for a null allele, but clear Mendelian inheritance was not demonstrated. These results led us to study the inheritance of C4 levels in normal families, and the results showed a strong heritability (about 50–65%) with some maternal influence, but the mechanism that determines the levels of C4 from these studies seems to be polygenic rather than simply Mendelian. However, it does not exclude the possibility that some low levels (half the normal values for example) may be inherited in simple Mendelian fashion (Figure 6.5).

Similarly, there are reports indicating that low C2 levels, possibly heterozygous C2-deficient individuals, are more frequent among rheumatological patients than among normal blood donors. On the other hand, a hypocomplementemic form of multiple sclerosis of genetic origin and characterized by low C3 or BF levels has also been reported by some investigators. Our own experience with this disease is

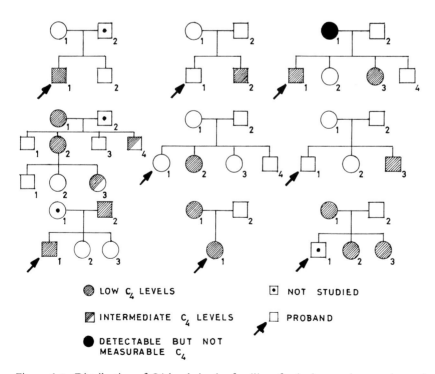

Figure 6.5. Distribution of C4 levels in the families of spinal muscular atrophy patients.

Table 6.2. Parent–child correlation coefficients for the
C4 levels.

	n	v	p
Son–father	16	0.302	0.128
Son–mother	19	0.540	0.009
Daughter–father	16	0.213	0.214
Daughter–mother	20	0.327	0.080
Child –father	28	0.273	0.080
Child –mother	31	0.444	0.006

rather contradictory, for in a sample of 104 multiple sclerosis patients from the North East of England, 'complement abnormalities' were not significantly different in number between patients and controls. Low complement levels of genetic origin have also been described recently in insulin-dependent diabetes (C4), in HLA-B8-positive patients with Graves' disease (C4), and in healthy individuals associated with the *HLA-Dw2* allele (C2 and C4).

Overall it seems clear that the low concentrations of the complement components may be due to a wide variety of factors. For instance they may be the expression of complement consumption or, if they are genetically controlled, they may be the result of:

1. Null alleles occurring at only one of the duplicated loci.
2. A genuine concentration-controlling gene.
3. The subclinical formation of immune complexes due to the production of low-affinity antibodies that is perhaps also under genetic control.

But many factors are known to be involved in the control of the levels of circulating proteins, and among them direct genetic control for some of the human complement components can neither be excluded nor confirmed.

Genetic deficiencies of complement components

Isolated complement deficiencies have now been described for almost all the complement components including C1r, C4, C2, C3, C5, C6, C7 and C8, for the C1 inhibitor and C3b inactivator, and for the Factor B. In all cases the transmission has been shown to be autosomal recessive except the C1 inhibitor deficiency which is inherited as autosomal dominant.

In general, these isolated complement deficiencies may, among other possibilities, be the outcome of genetically determined defects resulting from any one of the following:

1. Total absence of synthesis due to lack of function of either a structural or a regulator gene.

2. The production of a functionally inactive component due to a structural defect.

3. The continuous synthesis of a specific inhibitor as a result of de-repression of a regulator gene.

Three major clinical groups have been observed among patients with complement deficiencies.

The first, associated with C3 and C3b inactivator deficiencies, is a severe immune deficiency towards bacterial infections, very similar to that seen in antibody deficiency syndromes. The second is infection produced by *Neisseria gonorrhoeae* and *Neisseria meningitidis* and seen in patients with deficiencies of C4, C5, C7 and C8. The third is a strong association with systemic lupus erythematosus and a group of other immune complex/autoimmune diseases. They have been described in individuals lacking C1, C2, C4, C5 and C8. These associations may be due to an ascertainment effect, since these types of patients are usually studied for complement components: the liability to develop an immune complex/autoimmune disease may be a direct consequence of the complement deficiency; or it may be due to another gene (possibly an *Ir* gene) for which the complement deficiency is just a marker. It is not clear so far which of these mechanisms is responsible for the associations.

6.6. Complement receptors

The receptors for the complement components are becoming an interesting area of research with far wider implications than previously thought. Surface complement receptors have been observed on all leukocyte types, erythrocytes, platelets and mast cells, among others, and so far eight types have been described (Table 6.3).

The receptors so far studied have been shown to be single or double chain

Table 6.3. Specificity and physiological role of surface complement receptors so far described.

Receptor	Specificity	Physiological role
CR1	C3b, C4b, iC3b	Clearance of immune complexes
CR2	C3d-g, C3d	Regulation of T-cell activation
CR3	C3d-g, iC3b	Function in phagocytosis
C3a-R	C3a	Histamine release by the neutrophil
C5a-R	C5a	Induction of chemotaxis
C3e-R	C3e	Induction of leukocytosis
H-R	Factor H	Stimulation of superoxide metabolism in monocytes
C1q-R	C1q	Enhancement of neutrophil bacteriocidal activity

glycoproteins of varied molecular weights. The physiological role of CR1 seems to be the neutralization of soluble immune complexes. In fact, reduced numbers of CR1 have been found on the erythrocyte surface in patients with systemic lupus erythematosus and some of their relatives, suggesting Mendelian inheritance of this trait. The CR2 has only been found on B lymphocytes and is perhaps important in regulating T-cell activation. The other receptors seem to play various roles in the inflammatory response.

On the other hand, leukocytes have also been observed to express complement components on their surface and to be able to activate the complement system. These facts suggest that the overall function of the complement system is not only concerned with soluble proteins, but that it may be important as a regulator of cell-mediated immunity. If this were so, it would perhaps be the explanation for the preservation of coding for complement components within the MHC.

6.7. *Evolutionary aspects of the complement system*

The evolutionary aspects of the complement system are of interest. Questions raised are: first, how the system came to be the complex series of interrelated events that it is today? and, secondly, what genetic mechanisms were responsible for its diversification?

Physicochemically, three groups of similar components are found within the complement system. C2 and BF are not only coded within the HLA system, but are also similar in structure. C4 resembles C3 quite closely and also bears some resemblance to C5. Finally, C6 and C7 not only act in sequence, but also seem to be similar and closely linked to each other. These similarities can be explained, following Lachmann and Hobart, if one assumes that the original complement system was merely an amplification mechanism for which only two components, C3 and BF, would have been needed. This is the 'archaeo-complement' and corresponds to today's alternative pathway. It is then suggested that both the classical and terminal sequences arose by gene duplication from the alternative pathway.

Recent evidence has appeared regarding the linkage of three functionally related complement proteins in man: CR1, the C4-binding protein (C4-bp) and factor H. This gene cluster is not linked to the HLA system, but it is interesting that a membrane protein (CR1) is genetically linked to other related components, and also that many complement components are arranged in clusters that appeared to be preserved by evolution.

Bibliography

Alper, C. A., Genetics and the C3 molecule. *Vox Sang.*, **25**: 1 (1973).
Averill, B. K. and Bernal, J. E., Genetic and environmental influences on serum levels of human C4. *Ann. Hum. Biol.*, **11**: 149 (1984).

Awdeh, Z. L. and Alper, C. A., Inherited structural polymorphism of the fourth component of human complement. *Proc. Natl Acad. Sci. USA*, 17: 3576 (1980).

Bernal, J. E., Papiha, S. S., Keyeux, G., Lanchbury, J. S. and Mauff, G., Complement polymorphism in Colombia. *Ann. Hum. Biol.*, 12: 261 (1985).

Bronnestam, R., Studies of the C3 polymorphism. Relationship between phenotype and quantitative immunochemical measurements. *Hum. Hered.*, 23: 128 (1973).

Bronnestam, R., Studies of the C3 polymorphism. Relationship between phenotype and conversion rate *in vitro*. *Hum. Hered.*, 23: 220 (1973).

Bronnestam, R. and Cedergren, B., Studies of the C3 polymorphism. Relationship between C3 phenotypes and antibody titres. *Hum Hered.*, 23: 214 (1973).

Brunn-Petersen, G., Lamm, L. U., Jacobsen, B. K. and Kristensen, T., Genetics of complement C4. Two homoduplication haplotypes *C4S C4S* and *C4F C4F* in a family. *Hum. Genet.*, 61: 36 (82).

Campbell, R. D. and Porter, R. R., molecular cloning and characterisation of the gene coding for human complement protein factor B. *Proc. Natl Acad. Sci. USA*, 80: 4464 (1983).

Colten, H. R., Biosynthesis of the MHC-linked complement proteins (C2, C4 and factor B) by mononuclear phagocytes. *Mol. Immunol.*, 19: 1279 (1982).

Colten, H. R. and Einstein, L. P., Complement metabolism: cellular and humoral regulation. *Transplant. Rev.*, 32: 3 (1976).

Dierich, M. P., Scheiner, O., Mussel, H. H., Hamman, K. P., Schopf, R. E. and Schulz, T., Characterisation of complement receptors. *Mol. Immunol.*, 19: 1255 (1982).

Dykman, T. R., Hatch, J. A. and Atkinson, J. P., Polymorphism of the human C3b/C4b receptor. *J. Exp. Med.*, 159: 691 (1984).

Eiberg, H., Mohr, J., Staub Nielsen, L. and Simonsen, N., Genetics and linkage relationships of the C3 polymorphism: discovery of *C3–Se* linkage and assignment of *LES–C3–DM–Se–PEPD–Lu* synteny to chromosome 19. *Clin. Genet.*, 24: 159 (1983).

Fearon, D., Daha, M. R., Weiler, J. M. and Austen, K. F., The natural modulation of the amplification phase of complement activation. *Transplant. Rev.*, 32: 12 (1976).

Hauptmann, G., Sasportes, M., Tongio, M. M., Mayer, S. and Dausset, J., The localization of the *Bf* locus within the *MHS* region on chromosome No. 6. *Tissue Antigens*, 7: 52 (1976).

Hobart, M. J., Joysey, V. and Lachmann, P. J., Inherited structural variation and linkage relationship of C7. *J. Immunogenet.*, 5: 157 (1978).

Hobart, M. J., Vaz Guedes, M. A. and Lachmann, P. J., Polymorphism of human C5. *Ann. Hum. Genet.*, 45: 1 (1981).

Lachmann, P. J., Complement. In *The Antigens*, edited by M. Sela. Academic Press, New York (1977).

Lachmann, P. J. and Hobart, M. J., Complement genetics in relation to HLA. *Br. Med. Bull.*, 34: 247 (1978).

Marshall, W. H., Grandy, R. and Schroeder, M. L., The *C2* deficiency gene is allelic to *C2* structural genes. *Histocompatibility Testing*, p. 937. UCLA University Press, Los Angeles (1980).

Mauff, G., Bender, K. and Fischer, B., Genetic polymorphism of the fourth component of human complement. *Vox Sang.*, 34: 286 (1978).

Mauff, G., Bender, K., Giles, C. M., Goldman, S., Opferkuch, W. and Wachauf, B., Human C4 polymorphism: pedigree analysis of qualitative, quantitative and functional parameters as a basis for phenotype interpretations. *Hum. Genet.*, 65: 362 (1984).

Meo, T., Atkinson, J., Marietta, B., Bernoco, D. and Cepellini, R., Mapping of the HLA locus controlling C2 structural variants and linkage disequilibrium between alleles C2² and Bw15. *Eur. J. Immunol.*, 6: 916 (1976).

Meo, T., Atkinson, J. P., Bernoco, D. and Cepelllini, R., Structural heterogeneity of C2 complement protein and its genetic variants in man: a new polymorphism of the *HLA* region. *Proc. Natl Acad. Sci. USA*, **74**: 1672 (1977).

Ochs, H. D., Rosenfield, S. I., Thomas, E. D., Giblett, E. R., Alper, C. A., Dupont, B., Schaller, J. G., Gilliland, B. C., Hansen, J. A. and Wedgewood, R. J., Linkage between the gene (or genes) controlling synthesis of the fourth component of complement and the major histocompatibility complex. *N. Engl. J. Med.*, **296**: 470 (1977).

Ohayon, E., Mouson, A., Hauptmann, G., Klein, J. and Ducos, J., Genetic linkage between Bf S0.7 (Bf S1) and HLA-Bw50. *Hum. Genet.*, **54**: 417 (1980).

O'Neil, G. J. and Dupont, B., Serum C4 levels, Chido, Rodgers and allotypes of C4 component of complement. *Transplant. Proc.*, **11**: 1102 (1979).

Papiha, S. S., Bernal, J. E. and Mehrotra, M., Genetic polymorphism of serum proteins and levels of immunoglobulin and complement components in high caste community (Brahmins) of Madhya Pradesh, India. *Jap. J. Hum. Genet.*, **25**: 1 (1980).

Papiha, S. S., Bernal, J. E., Roberts, D. F., Habeebullah, C. M. and Mishra, S. C., C3 polymorphism in some Indian populations. *Hum. Hered.*, **29**: 193 (1979).

Petersen, G. B., Sorensen, I. J., Buskjaer, L. and Lamm, L. U., Genetic studies of complement C4 in man. *Hum. Genet.*, **53**: 31 (1976).

Rittner, C., Valentine-Thon, E., Bertrams, J., Gross-Wilde, H. and Schneider, M., Family Bromb.: *Bf* and *C4* gene cluster very close to *HLA-D(DR)*. In *Histocompatibility Testing*, p. 933. UCLA University Press, Los Angeles (1980).

Sorensen, H. and Dissing, J., C3 polymorphism in relation to age. *Hum. Hered.*, **25**: 284 (1975).

Steckel, E. W., York, R. G., Monahan, J. B. and Sodetz, J. M., The eighth component of human complement: purification and physiochemical characterisation of its unusual subunit structure. *J. Biol. Chem.*, **255**: 11997 (1980).

Sucia-Foca, N. and O'Neill, G., Families with C2° and C4 functional deficiencies. In *Histocompatibility Testing*, p. 938. UCLA University Press, Los Angeles (1980).

Sundsmo, J. S., The leukocyte complement system. *Fed. Proc.*, **41**: 3094 (1982).

Teisberg, P., High voltage agarose gel electrophoresis in the study of C3 polymorphism. *Vox. Sang.*, **19**: 47 (1970).

Teisberg, P., Olaisen, B., Jonassen, R., Gedde-Dahl, T. and Thorsby, E., The genetic polymorphism of the fourth component of human complement: methodological aspects and a presentation of linkage and association data relevant to its localisation in the HLA region. *J. Exp. Med.*, **146**: 1380 (1977).

Chapter 7. Genetics of the blood groups

The blood groups have a very special position in immunogenetics since it was through them that a series of important genetic principles was first demonstrated, while identification of blood groups is of overwhelming importance in daily clinical practice.

There is no systematic and organized nomenclature of the blood groups and their genes. The groups first discovered were identified alphabetically, but then usually each group was given the name of the first person in whom it was discovered (such as in Duffy and Kidd), while a part of this name came to be used to designate the genetic locus (*Fy* for Duffy and *Jk* for Kidd — the latter since the child in whom the Kidd system was discovered was J. Kidd). For the alleles there are three types of nomenclature in use:

letters as in *A* or *B* of the ABO system
capital and small letters as in the case of *Cc* or *Ee* in the rhesus system
a symbol with a superscript letter as in Lu^a and Lu^b

The following will describe some of the better-known blood groups, without attempting a comprehensive coverage, to provide a basis for the later discussion of the associations between blood groups and disease.

Table 7.1. Some of the blood-group systems.

System	First described by	Main antigens
ABO	Landsteiner	A1, A2, B, O, H, Ax, Am
Lewis	Mourant	Le^a, Le^b
MNSs	Landsteiner and Levine	M, N, S, s, M^g, M^k
P	Landsteiner and Levine	$P1, P2, P^k$
Rh	Landsteiner and Wiener	C, c, D, E, e, D^u
Duffy	Cutbush, Mollison and Parkin	Fy^a, Fy^b, Fy^x
Kell	Coombs, Mourant and Race	$K, k, Kp^a, Kp^b, Js^a, Js^b$
Lutheran	Callender, Race and Paykoc	Lu^a, Lu^b
Kidd	Allen, Diamond and Niedziela	Jk^a, Jk^b

Table 7.1 sets out the blood groups described here, with the name of the discoverer and the principal antigens.

7.1. *The ABO and related systems*

The ABO blood groups are determined by three alleles, *A*, *B* and *O*. Two of them, *A* and *B*, produce a characteristic antigen, while *O* does not and is therefore regarded as an amorphic gene. With these three genes there are six possible phenotypes (AA,AO, BB, BO, AB and OO), but the phenotypes AA and AO are indistinguishable by routine laboratory techniques, and so are BB and BO.

It is well known that the serum of a normal person contains antibodies which do not react with the antigens of the ABO system that he possesses. Type A individuals therefore have anti-B serum, while those in group B have anti-A. Obviously the individuals of type O can carry both anti-A and anti-B, while those of group AB have neither (Table 7.2).

The formation of the ABO blood groups and their antibodies is interesting. The blood groups derive from a precursor substance upon which acts the product of a gene (*H*) converting it to H substance; if this gene is not present, the precursor substance remains unchanged. The substance H is the substrate for the action of genes *A* and *B* which respectively convert it into antigen A or B. They leave unconverted a variable quantity of substance H. Individuals with no *A* or *B* genes (genotype *OO*), are obviously unable to convert substance H (Figure 7.1).

Table 7.2. Antigens and antibodies of the ABO system.

Phenotype	Genotype	Antigens on erythrocyte	Antibodies in serum
A	*A/A* *A/O*	A	Anti-B
B	*B/B* *B/O*	B	Anti-A
AB	*A/B*	A and B	None
O	*O/O*	None	Anti-A Anti-B

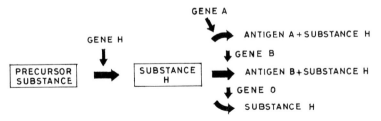

Figure 7.1. Diagram of the formation of A and B antigens from the precursor substance.

Anti-A and anti-B antibodies are produced early in life, by immunisation with substances from the environment similar to antigens A and B.

Secretor status

Besides the *A*, *B*, *O* and *H* genes, there are other genes which interact with them in the final formation of their products. It has been known for a long time that some people secrete in their saliva the antigens of their ABO blood group. Some individuals of blood group A have the A substance in their saliva and other body fluids while others do not. This peculiar situation behaves in a Mendelian fashion, with secretion being dominant over non-secretion and controlled by two alleles, *Se* (secretor) and *se* (non-secretor).

Another pair of alleles involved in secretor status are named *Yy*. Development of the A antigen depends upon the action of the *Y* gene. A very peculiar situation is observed in an individual with genotype *Yy* (extremely rare) who is also a secretor (*Se*) and blood group A. Such an individual secretes in his saliva the A antigen but this does not appear in his erythrocytes. While the Y system is therefore important in the production and secretion of the A antigens, it is not necessary for the normal production of B and H products.

Subgroups of A

There exist many variants of antigens A and B, although fewer of the latter. The most common subgroups of the antigen A are known as A1 and A2. Their biochemical differences are not clear. These two antigens are the products of two alleles and therefore what we term the *A* gene consists in reality of two classes, *A1* and *A2*.

Among the less frequent subgroups A3 is interesting, and is characterized by the partial agglutination by anti-A plus anti-B. This A3 subgroup is also genetically controlled apparently by an allele at the ABO locus. It is always necessary to distinguish it from a chimera, leukaemia and other peculiar situations in which the interaction between A2 and B can produce what seems to be A3.

There are two other weaker classes of A, known as A_x and A_m. The cells of both react with anti H. The cells of A_x individuals do not react with anti-A of B donors, but do so with anti-A derived from O donors. The cells of types A_m do not react with anti-A from either.

Anomalies of the ABO system

The Bombay phenotype is a very rare situation in which the cells of an individual do not react with anti-A, anti-B or anti-H, but his serum contains the three antibodies. These individuals are in fact homozygous for an inactive allele *h*, and do not therefore form the H substance, so there is no substrate on which the *A* and *B* gene products can act.

Acquired B antigen

Some individuals with blood group A can, by an unknown mechanism, absorb on to their erythrocytes a substance similar to the B antigen. This antigen may come from the polysaccharides of organisms such as *Escherichia coli* and *Proteus vulgaris*, which are well known to have similar properties to B antigens.

The Lewis system

This system is biochemically associated with ABO and secretor status. Its antigens are soluble in water and are chiefly present in saliva, although small quantities are observed in plasma and can also be absorbed on to the surface of the erythrocytes. It seems, therefore, that the antigens of the Lewis system are present only secondarily on the erythrocytes.

The expression of these antigens is controlled by several genes, which interact with those of the *ABO, H* and secretor systems, which are independently inherited and which act in sequence; first the Lewis, then the *H* genes, then the secretor and finally the *ABO* genes. The Lewis system is defined genetically by the alleles *Le* and *le*.

Biochemical basis of the expression of the Lewis and ABO (H) substances

A very important point, that helps in understanding the biochemical basis of the expression of the ABO (H) and Lewis substances, is that the genes which control these blood groups do not code for their immunological specificities but for an enzyme which controls the addition of a given sugar to a precursor substance. In this sense, the antigenic determinants of the ABO and Lewis blood groups are secondary genetic products, the primary ones being the enzymes responsible for the addition of the sugar.

As primary genetic products, the gene *A* produces a transferase, *N*-acetyl-galactosamine, the gene *B* a galactosyltransferase, and the *H* and *Le* genes two distinct types of fucosyltransferase. The gene *Se* does not produce an enzyme, but is necessary for the production of the fucosyltransferase coded for by gene *H*, although this effect occurs only in certain organs.

The secondary genetic products (that is the antigenic determinants) of the ABO and Lewis groups are very similar, consisting of glycoproteins or glycolipids which contain numerous chains of oligosaccharides of at least five sugars: D-galactose, L-fucose, *N*-acetyl-D-glucosamine, *N*-acetyl-D-galactosamine and sialic acid. To produce the antigenic determinants, the primary genetic products interact with a precursor substance that can be of two types: type 1 is an oligosaccharide and contains β-galactosyl-*N*-acetylglucosamine with the two sugars linked 1 → 3; type 2 is the same oligosaccharide which contains the same unit but with the sugars linked 1 → 4.

If the precursor substance has both types of chain, the genes *ABO* and *Lewis*

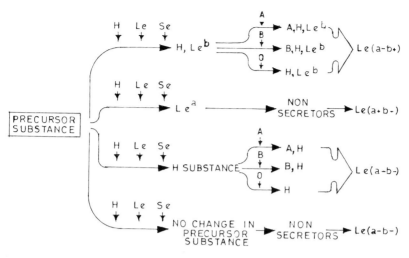

Figure 7.2. Interaction between *Le*, *H*, *Se* and *ABO* genes.

act upon it to produce the transfer of a specific substance giving the final structure of antigenic determinant. For instance, the product of gene *H* (the fucosyltransferase) controls the addition of L-fucose to the type 1 chain to produce the antigenic structure of the active Le^a substance. When the two genes *H* and *Le* are present, there are two substitutions of L-fucose to give the final stucture of the Le^b specificity, but the addition of one of them needs an L-fucosyltransferase that has been observed only in the milk of secretor individuals of blood groups A, B and H. The interaction of these genes occurs in such a way that the expression of one of them is dependent upon the presence of the other gene, and this quite common finding in blood groups is known as epistasis.

Figure 7.2 shows the interaction between the genes *Le*, *H*, *Se* and *ABO* to give the final secreted product in the saliva and the Lewis phenotype of the erythrocytes. It can be seen that there is a clear association between secretor status and the Lewis phenotype, as is to be expected from the mechanism of epistasis. Therefore all individuals *Le* (a^-b^+) are secretors, those *Le* (a^+b^-) are non-secretors and those *Le* (a^-b^-) can be secretors or non-secretors.

7.2. *The MN and Ss groups*

The MN blood groups were first detected in 1927. The system is controlled by a pair of alleles which appear to determine the final antigens of the groups M and N. There are therefore three genotypes *MM*, *MN* and *NN* with the corresponding phenotypes M, MN and N.

The alleles *S* and *s*, closely linked with *M* and *N*, are also alleles to a third one

S^U, which is most common in Negroes and is also present in individuals who have neither S nor s. The erythrocytes for the majority of these individuals do not agglutinate with anti-U (an antibody which does not agglutinate the cells of 1% of Negroes) and there seems to be a mixture of anti-S and anti-s. There are, however, exceptions in a few individuals who have neither S nor s but are U-positive.

The immunochemical basis of the MN system is as complex as that of the ABO and Lewis blood groups. It has been proposed that the final antigenic formation of this system is achieved in a similar way to that of the ABO groups, but by the addition of neuraminyl groups. But it has also been proposed that the antigen N is a precursor substance upon which the genes N and M act. By this mechanism the gene N would have to be an amorph and would therefore leave intact the antigen N. The gene M would convert only part of the antigen N to antigen M in the heterozygous state, but would convert it all in the homozygous state.

There are also less frequent antigens in the MNSs system. The gene M^g produces small quantities of M and a larger quantity of N. The M^k M^v, Mt^a and M^c, although rare as antigens, may be more frequent as natural antibodies.

7.3. *The P system*

This was discovered during the experiments which led to the discovery of the antigens of the MN system. When human cells were injected into rabbits, the antibodies produced agglutinated the red cells of more than 70% of the population studied. The agglutinated erythrocytes were therefore designated P-positive and the others P-negative.

Later it was shown that a rare antibody already described (anti-Jay or Tj^a) was also part of the P system. There are therefore three alleles in the P system, today known as P^1 (formerly giving the P-positive phenotype), P^2 (formerly giving the P-negative homozygotes) and p (formerly the allele Tj^a). Similar to what is observed in the ABO groups, almost every P^2 individual has anti-P^1 in his serum. The biochemistry of the P system was clarified by the discovery of a very rare variant among Finns, called P^k. P^k individuals have serum antibodies which react with P^1 and P^2 but not with p or other P^k cells. The P^k antigen has been identified as a ceramide trihexoside, while the P^2 antigen is a glycosphingolipid globoside. In consequence, it has been proposed that the products coded for by the P genes are enzymes of the transferase type that catalyse successive transformation until the final product is obtained (the antigen P). This process can be explained in two ways: either the genes P^k and P^1 are closely linked and both produce a galactosyltransferase necessary for the production of the antigens P^k and P^1, or the gene P^k produces the transferase and the gene P^1 produces a regulator molecule that acts upon the transferase, enabling it to produce the antigens P^1 and P^k.

7.4. The Rh group

From the purely clinical point of view this system is more important than those
outlined above, because it is the main cause of haemolytic disease of the newborn.
However, its chemical structure is not yet completely determined and the genetic
mechanisms and the nomenclature of this system remain controversial. Two
mechanisms have been postulated: one suggests that the expression of these antigens depends upon three closely linked loci, while the other postulates a single
multi-allelic locus.

In 1940 an antibody was described which was produced by immunizing rabbits
with the blood of the rhesus monkey, which also reacted with the blood of 85%
of the human population, and which was not related to the ABO, MN or P blood
groups. This antibody was called Rh. With the discovery soon afterwards of other
specificities associated with Rh, this was called D (or Rh$^+$), and the newer ones C,
c, E and e. The products C, c at one locus and E, e at another are allelic forms and
cannot therefore be inherited from the same parent.

Fisher later proposed that the mechanism of heredity of the Rh system was
based on eight allelic combinations (CDE, CDe, Cde, CdE, cDE, cDe, cdE and
cde), which are inherited as haplotypes, each letter indicating the genetic determination of a given specific determinant. Each individual therefore has two
haplotypes for Rh, one coming from the father and the other from the mother;
the genotype is the expression of both of them. The most frequent haplotypes in
the European population are CDe (approximately 40%), cde (39%) and cDE
(14%). The majority of Rh-negative individuals are cde/cde. Wiener proposed
that there was a single locus controlling the expression of the whole Rh system,
and used a different nomenclature with r indicating the rhesus negative gene, R
the rhesus positive, and a series of superscripts for the others. The terms employed
in both systems for the Rh haplotypes are summarised in Table 7.3.

The genetic basis of the Rh system is still under discussion. For some time the
opinion of Fisher was accepted on the existence of three linked loci, but the extraordinary number of known specificities is difficult to explain according to this

Table 7.3. Nomenclature of the Rh
system.

Fisher	Wiener
CDE	R^z
CDe	R^1
cDE	R^2
cde	r
Cde	r'
cdE	r''
CdE	r^Y

mechanism and the other multiple allele systems that have since been discovered (e.g., Gm) lend support to the single-locus hypothesis. The genes which determine the Rh system are located on chromosome number 1.

Variants of the Rh system

Variants have been described for each one of the antigenic determinants of the Rh system. The most important, D^u, is common in Negroes and can stimulate the production of antibodies (anti-D) in a Rh^- (dd) person.

Another important variant is the *null Rh*, in which there are no antigens of the Rh system. This situation may be present when an individual is homozygous for the amorph r (- - -) or when an individual is a homozygote for a suppressor gene ($X^o r$) which is independent of the Rh system and which may also express itself by inhibiting antigens of other systems, particularly MNSs.

Other antigens

The antigen Lw was so named for Landsteiner and Wiener, its describers. It was once thought to be part of the Rh system, but today is established that they are independently inherited, although both products (Lw and CDE) may originate from the same substrate.

The Duffy system consists essentially of alleles Fy^a, Fy^b and Fy. There are four possible phenotypes

Phenotypes	Genotypes
Fy (a + b +)	$Fy^a Fy^b$
Fy (a + b -)	$Fy^a Fy^a$ or $Fy^a Fy$
Fy (a - b +)	$Fy^b Fy^b$ or $Fy^b Fy$
Fy (a - b -)	$FyFy$

This last phenotype, Fy (a - b -), very common in Negroes, but extremely rare in whites, is the product of a third allele called *Fy*. It seems that there are two forms of this allele: one does not produce either Fy^a or Fy^b, and the other reacts weakly with some antisera for Fy^b, the latter is called Fy^x.

In the Kell system it is possible that the genetic mechanism controlling the synthesis of the products is very similar to that of Rh, determined by either several alleles at a single locus or by various loci closely linked together. In Kell three pairs of alleles have been identified named K/k, Kp^a/Kp^b and Js^a/Js^b. However, at least 18 antigens in this system are known, some of them not very well defined, for example, the antigens Williams, McLeod and Closs.

The Lutheran system, like the Duffy, consists of two alleles, Lu^a and Lu^b, and three principal phenotypes.

Phenotypes	Genotype
Lu (a + b +)	$Lu^a Lu^b$
Lu (a + b -)	$Lu^a Lu^a$
Lu (a - b +)	$Lu^b Lu^b$

There is, however, a fourth extremely rare phenotype, Lu (a – b –), attributable to recessivity of an extremely rare gene, or to the presence of another gene which inhibits the expression of the genes of the Lutheran system. The locus of the Lutheran system is linked with that of secretor status; this was the first case of autosomal linkage described in man.

The Kidd blood group has two principal alleles, Jk^a and Jk^b, while a third allele, Jk, is responsible for the phenotype Jk (a – b –). The only blood-group system on the X chromosome in man is called Xg. Since Xg^a is dominant over Xg, the phenotype Xg(a +) is more frequent in women than in men, for in women it includes the heterozygotes Xg^aXg, whereas in men the frequencies of the phenotypes are those of the genes.

Of the many other antigenic systems of the erythrocytes, it is worth mentioning the Goodspeed (DBG), since one of its antigens (BG^a) is related to HLA-B7 of the major histocompatibility system. The relationship is not very clear, but it seems that the antigen BG^a is the portion of HLA-B7 that survived to the maturation of the erythrocytes. Recently, similar relationships have been observed between BG^b and HLA-Bw17 and between BG^c and HLA-A28.

Bibliography

Dodd, B. E. and Lincoln, P. J., *Blood Group Topics*. Arnold, London (1975).

Fudenberg, H. H., Pink, J. R. L., Wang, A. and Douglas, S. D., *Basic Immunogenetics*. Oxford University Press, New York (1978).

Giblett, E., *Genetic Markers in Human Blood*. F. A. Davis, Philadelphia (1969).

Grollman, E. F., Kobata, A. and Ginsburg, V., An enzymatic basis for Lewis blood types in man. *J. Clin. Invest.*, 48: 1489 (1969).

Harris, H., *The Principles of Biochemical Genetics*. North Holland, Amsterdam (1980).

Kabat, E. A., *Structural Concepts in Immunology and Immunochemistry*. Holt, Rinehart and Winston, New York (1976).

Kabat, E. A., *Blood Group Substances: Their Chemistry and Immunochemistry*. Academic Press, New York (1956).

Morgan, W. T., A contribution to human biochemical genetics: the chemical basis of blood group specificity. *Proc. R. Soc. Lond. [Biol.]*, 151: 308 (1960).

Mourant, A. E., Kopec, A. D. and Domaniewska-Sobczac, K., *The Distribution of the Human Blood Groups and Other Polymorphisms*. Oxford University Press, Oxford (1976).

Pollack, M. S., Crawford, M. N., Robinson, H. M., Berger, R., Sabo, B. and O'Neill, G. J., Bg^b expression in relation to the HLA-B17 antigen splits BW57 and BW58 and the cross-reactions of anti-Bg^b antibodies. *Vox Sang.*, 43: 1 (1982).

Race, R. R. and Sanger, R., *Blood Groups in Man*. Blackwell, Oxford (1975).

Walker, M. E., Rubistein, P. and Allen, F. H., Biochemical genetics of MN. *Vox Sang.*, 32: 111 (1977).

Watkins, W. M., Blood group substances. *Science*, 152: 172 (1966).

PART II

CLINICAL APPLICATIONS

Chapter 8. Immunodeficiencies

Clinical investigation has made good use of nature's experiments for understanding the immunodeficiencies. This chapter reviews the more common defects of T and B cells, and later chapters deal with defects of the complement and phagocytic systems. Medical treatments will be briefly indicated, but those that refer to tissue transplantation will be explained conceptually in the chapter on transplants. We will deal first with the pure B-cell defects, T cells, combined deficiencies and others. Figure 8.1 summarizes the mechanisms that may lead to immunodeficiencies.

8.1. Primary disorders of B cells

General considerations

The usual clinical presentation of the patient with primary deficiency of B cells is obviously recurrent infections, particularly by *Haemophilus influenzae*, *Staphylococcus aureus* or *Diplococcus pneumoniae*, although any infection due to a non-pathogenic agent should be investigated as a possible manifestation of an underlying immunodeficiency. In any case, immunodeficiencies are not always clearly symptomatic at an early age; sinusitis in these cases is the predominant symptom. Among cutaneous manifestations, an eczema that is difficult to manage is seen occasionally; when associated with allergies and recurrent abcesses of the skin this should direct attention to the possibility of the hyper-immunoglobulin E syndrome, which will be dealt with in detail later.

In primary disorders of B cells, gastrointestinal symptoms are also common and may even be the reason for consultation. While malabsorption symptomatology is not seen very often, infections by *Giardia lamblia* are common. A high incidence of pernicious anaemia is also observed in these patients.

Autoimmunity and malignancy in immunodeficiency

Patients with immunoglobulin deficiencies, and their families, have a high incidence of autoimmune disease. The mechanism to explain this association is not known. Similarly, it has been calculated that in patients with immunodeficiencies

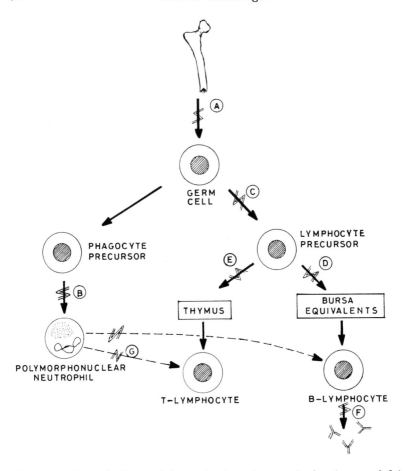

Figure 8.1. General scheme of the mechanisms that may lead to immunodeficiency.

the incidence of malignant tumours is ten thousand times that in the general population. This is seen not only in natural immunodeficiencies but also in patients receiving immunosuppressors, which would support Burnett's theory of immunological surveillance, according to which the immune system surveys, controls and finally eliminates any tumoral manifestations as they appear. As yet, the mechanism to account for the association between immunodeficiency and malignancy is not established.

Classification of the B-cell disorders

The entities usually classified as mainly or totally due to dysfunction of B cells (Table 8.1) include the deficiency or absence of all the immunoglobulins, as well

Table 8.1. Disorders due to B-cell dysfunction.

Bruton-type agammaglobulinaemia
Variable common immunodeficiency
Selective deficiencies
IgE defects
Subgroup deficiencies
Transcobalamin deficiency

as selective deficiency of one of them and the defects of hypo- and hyper-immunoglobulin E.

General concepts of pathogenesis

It is clear that, given the complexity of the immune system, a defect in the production of antibodies may be due to a block at very different levels, from the formation of the B cells up to the synthesis of the immunoglobulin. The most important of these blocks may occur at the following levels (Figure 8.2):

1. early failure in the maturation of the B cells, leading to their absence;
2. failure of the switch mechanism of IgM–IgG–IgA–IgE;
3. incapacity to receive or process antigenic signals, although capable of producing antibodies;
4. excess in immunological suppressor mechanisms.

Let us examine these four points in more detail:

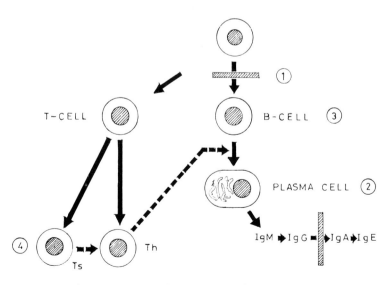

Figure 8.2. Blocks that may lead to a B-cell defect.

Absence of B cells

Unfortunately, the mechanisms of production of B cells from multipotential precursors are unknown, and this makes it difficult to indicate the precise sites at which their development may be blocked. Patients have been observed with panhypogamma-globulinaemia in which there are either no B lymphocytes or the number is very diminished, suggesting that the defect may lie in the induction of the maturation of these lymphocytes.

Failure of the switch mechanisms

This mechanism is important in the development of the B lymphocyte. A block in this process of differentiation will obviously lead to a dysgammaglobulinaemia with high levels of the immunoglobulins before the block.

Failure in the receptor mechanism of antigenic signals

It is believed that this block may be responsible for some of the forms of agamma-globulinaemia, as well as ataxia telangiectasia and some cases of selective deficiency of IgA.

Excess of suppressor mechanisms

In patients with the common variable type of hypogammaglobulinaemia the presence has been noted of suppressor T cells that can inhibit the synthesis of immunoglobulins *in vitro*; the pathogenic importance of this observation is not clear.

The delineation of these general concepts of the pathogenesis of the immunodeficiencies of B cells is of importance not so much in clarifying the etiology of the disorders, but more in demonstrating their great heterogeneity and the necessity of more detailed observations that may allow a better physiopathological classification. Nevertheless, several clinical pictures can be defined.

8.2. Bruton-type agammaglobulinaemia

This is the classic agammaglobulinaemia, inherited in an X-linked recessive form. As its name indicates, these patients have absence of immunoglobulins, but their cellular immune function is normal. Its true incidence is unknown, but in the UK it is approximately one case per hundred thousand individuals.

Anatomicopathological examination shows that germ cells and plasma cells are usually absent from the lymphoid tissue, the follicular structure is absent in the amygdala and Peyer plates, but the thymus is normal.

Although the total levels of circulating lymphocytes are normal in these patients, no B cells are found in blood or bone marrow. On the other hand, intracytoplasmic IgM has been observed in some of them, as well as a detectable but low level of circulating IgG, suggesting that the block may be subsequent to the formation of the precursors of the B cells. There is also evidence that some of these patients may have a defect in the receptor mechanism of the helper function of the B cells. This may be the mechanism which leads to immunodeficiency, since the B cells of these patients do not differentiate when they come in contact with T cells of normal individuals. For some time is was also thought that the pathogenic mechanism lay in the existence of T cells capable of suppressing the differentiation of B cells of the patients. However, it has been observed recently that elimination of the T cells is not followed by spontaneous differentiation of B cells, so that the role of these suppressor T cells in agammaglobulinaemia is not yet clear.

Clinical manifestations

The disease usually presents in the newborn when the levels of IgG derived from the mother drop to their lowest level; this occurs at about five to six months of age. As already mentioned, the usual symptoms are infective, particularly otitis, bronchitis, pneumonia, dermatitis or meningitis. The age of presentation and the persistence of the infectious symptomatology varies, and the first clinical manifestation may indeed be very late.

Although in general there are no symptoms of cell-mediated pathology, cases have been described with massive viral infection, suggesting that some of these patients may be extremely susceptible to certain viral diseases, particularly enteroviruses.

Diagnosis

In the classical form of the disease there is absence, or diminution in level, of the immunoglobulins, absence of B cells in peripheral blood, marked reduction of the B-dependent area of the lymphatic nodes, but intact cellular immunity.

The total levels of immunoglobulins are usually below 200 mg/100 ml, mostly made up of IgG; it is the other immunoglobulins that are either extremely low or absent. Exceptionally there may be absence of all immunoglobulins except IgE, the level of which is normal.

Biopsy of lymphatic nodes is not usually necessary, although it is very informative; intestinal biopsy may be of more help, since in some cases the complete absence of plasma cells from the lamina propria would establish the diagnosis.

Other examinations that may be helpful are the X-rays of frontal sinuses, paranasal sinuses and thorax at regular intervals, which allow the clinical course of the symptomatic patient to be followed at these levels. However, pulmonary function tests may also be useful, as well as the investigation of *Giardia lamblia* in patients with gastrointestinal symptoms.

Differential diagnosis

There may be problems in the differential diagnosis when there is prolonged physiological hypogammaglobulinaemia of the newborn. The diagnosis may not be established immediately and may require measurement of immunoglobulins at intervals of three months. A gradual increase in their levels argues against the congenital form.

If the severity of the immunological depression requires the administration of gammaglobulin before the diagnosis is established, these two entities may be differentiated by the increase of IgM and IgA in the course of time, since the commercial forms of gammaglobulin contain only small quantities of these two immunoglobulins.

In some countries, pronounced diminution in immunoglobulins may be due to severe enteropathy with protein loss through the gastrointestinal tract. In such cases, albumin determination and intestinal biopsy would allow the establishment of the differential diagnosis.

Treatment

Treatment of the primary humoral deficiencies is still not satisfactory, since it is oriented to the replacement of the deficit of immunoglobulins by gammaglobulin or fresh plasma and not to the correction of the primary immune defect.

Commercially available gammaglobulins contain some 150 mg of protein per ml, principally in the form of IgG. The half-life of this immunoglobulin in normal subjects is 20 days, but is very variable in agammaglobulinaemic patients, in whom there may be loss of protein through the gastrointestinal tract. There are various modes of treatment. Gammaglobulin can be administered subcutaneously or intramuscularly in doses of 0.6 ml/kg body weight, repeated every three to four weeks. Some patients may require it more often, perhaps weekly, to maintain the levels above 200 mg/100 ml.

Many of these patients develop systemic reactions to the gammaglobulin, not IgE mediated but possibly due to the formation of IgG aggregates, which activate the complement system and manifest as facial oedema, nausea, vomiting, abdominal pain and respiratory symptoms. The hyper-immune gammaglobulin that is prepared from normal donors with a high titre of specific antibodies has been very useful in reducing the severity of the attacks in immunodeficient patients exposed to varicella (Zoster immunoglobulin, ZIG).

As an alternative to gammaglobulin, the intravenous administration of fresh plasma has been used. This has four advantages over the usual treatment with gammaglobulin:

1. High levels of immunoglobulins are obtained more rapidly.
2. All the immunoglobulin classes are given.
3. There is no proteolysis by muscular enzymes.

4. Donors can be immunized in order to obtain high titres of specific antibodies.

The disadvantages of the administration of fresh plasma are the same as with any transfusion, such as serum hepatitis, transmission of cytomegalovirus, and transfusion reactions. To reduce the risk of hepatitis only one or two donors should be used, preferably from the family of the patient and negative for Australia antigen.

The recommended doses of plasma lie between 10 and 20 ml/kg body weight at intervals of two to four weeks, obviously while monitoring the levels of immunoglobulin of the patient.

8.3. Common variable immunodeficiency

General considerations

This type of immunodeficiency is less easy to define than the Bruton-type agammaglobulinaemia, and is more of the nature of a group of disorders in which the clinical manifestations and the immunological defects vary from patient to patient and even from time to time in a single patient.

The majority of these patients have a normal number of B lymphocytes, but some or all of these lymphocytes may not differentiate into plasma cells when exposed to an antigen. Although this group of defects is usually classified among those of B cells, little is known of the pathogenesis which may also involve T cells and macrophages. Various immunological mechanisms have been suggested to explain the pathogenesis of this varied group. Deficiency of helper T cells is one of them, since it has been observed that the B cells of some of these patients respond to antigenic stimulation by pokeweed when in contact with T cells of normal individuals. The reverse mechanism has also been observed: the lymphocytes of individuals with common variable immunodeficiency and normal B lymphocytes suppress the differentiation to plasma cells of antigenically stimulated normal lymphocytes, and the resulting excess in the suppressor mechanisms could lead to the immunodeficiency. However, macrophages are indispensable in T-cell activation and there may also be a deficiency at this level. There are observations of abnormalities in T-cell subsets in this as well as other immunodeficiencies. Thirteen patients recently studied with this type of deficiency showed a reduction of T_h lymphocytes ($T4^+$) while T_s cells ($T8^+$) were increased. An inversion of the normal ratio of T_h/T_s cells was also found in some of these patients. It seems that these abnormalities are common to other immunodeficiencies besides the common variable type. Another recent study of nine patients showed a reduction in the proliferative response of T-cell-enriched populations in most of them, suggesting a defect at the level of the macrophage-T cell interaction.

This group is also heterogeneous from the genetic point of view. In the majority of the patients there is no evidence of parent–child transmission, but some are clearly inherited as autosomal recessives.

Clinical manifestations

These are very similar to those of the congenital Bruton-type agammaglobulin-aemia, but usually present later, between 15 and 30 years of age. The auto-immune diseases have been particularly associated with this type of deficiency, particularly lupus erythematosus, rheumatoid arthritis, haemolytic anaemia and pernicious anaemia. An interesting observation is that pernicious anaemia is also associated with other immune defects as well as diabetes mellitus, whose immuno-genetic characteristics are just beginning to be understood. A recent report of common variable immunodeficiency in 30 children calls attention to its presence also at an early age. The age at diagnosis in children varies between 6 months and 15 years, the majority of them being diagnosed at around 10 years of age. Upper and lower respiratory tract infections are the most frequently observed of the infectious manifestations, recurrent pneumonia being the most severe complication. The immunological findings in children are very similar to those observed in adults, and a high proportion of the cases (27%) had a previous family history of immunodeficiency.

Diagnosis

Logically, immunoglobulin levels should be low as in the Bruton-type disease, usually less than 300 mg/100 ml, mostly of IgG. The number of B lymphocytes may be normal or slightly low. Cell-mediated immunity is normal or sometimes depressed, tests of delayed hypersensitivity are negative, and there is also diminution in the number of T cells. In these patients there may be important attendant complications. Thoracic X-rays may show chronic pulmonary disease. When there is an associated malabsorption syndrome, a test of absorption of *d*-xylose may give abnormal results. In these patients the appearance of signs and symptoms of auto-immune disease or of malignancy should be monitored.

Differential diagnosis

The differential diagnosis of the common variable immunodeficiency is carried out as in the Bruton type of agammaglobulinaemia, but the treatment of both is identical so this presents no clinical problems. It should also be differentiated from an enteropathic loss of protein in the cases associated with malabsorption. Serum albumin determinations are useful in these cases.

Treatment

The treatment is identical to that mentioned for agammaglobulinaemia, with gammaglobulin or fresh plasma. These patients usually require various continuous combinations of antibiotics that should be chosen according to the type of infection. Problems of intestinal absorption with enzymic deficit should be handled with adequate diet. In the cases of concomitant auto-immune disease, there may be a serious problem since the treatment with steroids makes these patients even more susceptible to bacterial infection.

8.4. *Selective deficiency of immunoglobulin M*

General considerations

A diagnosis of selective deficiency of IgM should be considered when the levels of this immunoglobulin are more than two standard deviations below the mean of the normal values for age, but where the levels of IgG and IgA are normal, and the functions of the T cells, macrophages and complement are intact. This deficiency may be of two types: either of genetic origin, or secondary to other defects, usually malignancies. As a primary defect, this deficiency is the second most frequent of the selective deficiencies, with an incidence of approximately one per thousand of the normal population.

The basic defect is unknown. All the patients so far seen have shown B lymphocytes with IgM on their surface, suggesting that the defect is at the level of the secretion of the immunoglobulin.

Clinical manifestations

The majority of these patients have increased susceptibility to infection, but others who are totally asymptomatic are not rare. We have observed a case in the mother of a child with spinal muscular atrophy, who seems to be otherwise totally normal. In the patients with bacterial symptomatology, a marked tendency is found towards rapid sepsis by a haematogenic mechanism, leading to death if aggressive antibiotic therapy is not instituted. There are two usual characteristics of these patients. The majority have splenomegaly and there is a high incidence of allergic pathology.

Treatment

Replacement therapy in IgM deficiency is not possible, since there is no commercial preparation of IgM, and it has a very short half-life (five days), so that fresh plasma cannot be used. The only viable tactic in these patients is the administration of antibiotics at the first sign of infection and a family study to detect deficiencies in other family members.

8.5. *Selective deficiency of immunoglobulin A*

General considerations

Selective deficiency of IgA is defined by levels lower than 5 mg/100 ml, with IgG and IgM normal and intact T-cell function. However, recent data indicate that many of these patients have accompanying defects of T cells of varying intensity. The management and prognosis of these patients obviously depends upon the degree of compromise of the cellular arm of the immune system.

From the purely pathogenic point of view, at least two entities are known. In one, the thymus has an important role and there may be a failure in activity of helper cells that would normally have been involved in the production of IgA. In the other form, the mechanism seems to be a failure of the terminal cellular differentiation of B lymphocytes. There is also a report of a case in which there was a failure in the assembly of heavy and light chains of IgA. More recently, a low-molecular-weight IgM was found in more than 30% of the patients with selective IgA deficiency, constituting up to 17% of the total circulating IgM. Immune complexes and associated diseases were more frequent in the IgA-deficient individuals with low-molecular-weight IgM, suggesting that the latter may be involved in the development of auto-immune concomitant pathology via the formation of immune complexes.

This type of deficiency is heterogeneous, clinically and etiologically, and its genetic basis is also variable. Selective deficiencies of IgA which were transmitted as autosomal dominants and autosomal recessives have been described. Moreover, the deficiency of this immunoglobulin is also observed in families of patients with panhypogammaglobulinaemia suggesting that there may be some etiological similarity between these two types of defects. It has also been described in patients with anomalies of chromosome 18, although the importance of this association is not yet clear. It is possibly more frequent than the deficiency of IgM, occurring in between 1 in 500 and 1 in a 1000 individuals in the general population. A recent study in Iceland confirmed its high incidence but also showed this deficiency to be associated with HLA-B8 as well as the phenotypes C4AQO and C3F of the complement system.

Clinical manifestations

Normal individuals are also observed with this deficiency, although a retrospective study of the clinically 'normal' ones shows associations with a significant pathology, so perhaps such individuals are not really 'normal'. In those who show symptoms, these relate to the organs in which IgA is the primary line of defence — the bronchopulmonary and gastrointestinal tracts. Besides recurrent infection, there have been observed allergies and pulmonary haemosiderosis as important pathologies of the respiratory tract. Infectious pathology is usually more of the viral than of the bacterial type. A factor which may be important in the manifestation of pulmonary disease is the level of IgE, for it has been observed that combined deficiency of IgE and IgA produces a less severe respiratory pathology than when there are normal or high levels of IgE but deficiency of IgA. This implies a modulating effect of IgA on IgE, which was also suggested in our study of immunoglobulin levels in normal populations; in populations exposed to greater antigenic stimulation, the levels of IgE and IgG increase while those of IgA decrease, possibly by a mechanism of common genetic control (see Chapter 3). On the other hand, the gastrointestinal manifestations are wider and include pernicious anaemia, coeliac disease and chronic diarrhoea. Those patients with coeliac disease also show a series of interesting immunological peculiarities. Three of these patients had an antibody that reacts with the basal membrane of the glomeruli; this was interpreted by the authors as possibly due to the absence of IgA in the intestinal epithelium, an absence which would allow the free passage of animal proteins that may cross-react with human proteins. Intestinal biopsy in these patients showed increased numbers of IgM-producing cells, possibly as a compensatory mechanism. However, the majority of patients with coeliac disease are not IgA deficient, and therefore the importance of this deficiency in the development of the disease is not established. There is, however, a very special predisposition, since the incidence of coeliac disease in IgA-deficient individuals is 12 times greater than in the general population.

Other types of pathology are also particularly associated with selective deficiency of IgA. In the literature, more than 70 cases have been reported of association between deficiency of IgA and auto-immune disease, almost half of them having symptoms of rheumatoid arthritis. There is also a high incidence of malignancy in this immunodeficiency especially of carcinomas of the gastrointestinal and the bronchopulmonary tracts, and of thymomas and reticulocellular sarcomas. These associations have been explained by a failure in the barrier of defence given by IgA, which allows the uncontrolled entrance of antigens to the circulatory stream, but other factors such as infection, genetics, and possibly defects of T cells, and formation of immune complexes, may be important in this respect.

Diagnosis

Usually in these patients there is no IgA in the serum or in the body secretions, but in the latter there may indeed be normal values. Cellular immunity may also be normal, including the tests of delayed hypersensitivity. The numbers of T and B lymphocytes are usually within normal limits. In cases of autoimmunity, auto-antibodies should be looked for.

Differential diagnosis

The isolated form should be differentiated from those associated with more severe pathology, although in some cases, as in ataxia telangiectasia in children, this is not always easy.

Treatment

There is still no adequate treatment for this type of immunodeficiency, other than purely symptomatic. Replacement therapy with gammaglobulin is contraindicated because of the risk of developing anti-IgA antibodies that could lead to later anaphylactoid reactions.

8.6. *IgE disorders*

There are two types of disorder of IgE which are associated with clinical pathology, the syndromes of hypo- and hyperimmunoglobulinaemia E. The definition of the second type is obvious, but that of hypogammaglobulinaemia E is more difficult unless there is clearly a frank deficiency. The normal levels of IgE have been defined as lying between 17.5 and 2177 i.u./ml, but our experience in more than 3000 specimens from various parts of the world indicates that less than 17.5 and indeed less than 10.5 i.u./ml is a common finding which is difficult to interpret as a deficiency, while levels of 1500 i.u./ml or more are rarely found in Caucasians but are frequent in tropical populations. Environmental variations are therefore important in deciding what are elevated levels. An adequate definition of deficiency seems to be levels below 7.5 i.u./ml.

Little is known about the rest of the immune system in these defects of IgE. The synthesis of this immunoglobulin is, like IgA, partially dependent on the thymus in two ways; it requires helper T cells for its initiation, and suppressor T cells for the control of the response. This mechanism explains the high levels of IgE found in some cellular immunodeficiencies since there is a sufficient number of T cells to initiate the synthesis but not to control it. The immunodeficiencies that occur with high levels of IgE are listed in Table 8.2.

Table 8.2. Immunodeficiencies associated with high IgE levels.

Wiskott-Aldrich syndrome
Di George's syndrome
Nezelof's syndrome
Selective deficiency of IgA
Syndrome of hyperimmunoglobulin E

Syndromes of hyperimmunoglobulin E

The clinical picture of these syndromes is very variable. However, it is important to emphasize that the syndrome of hyperimmunoglobulin E is in itself very rare; it does not include simply those patients with atopic eczema, high levels of IgE and repetitive skin infections. There are invariably episodes of severe furunculosis, and pneumonia principally due to *Staphylococcus aureus*, although *Haemophilus influenzae*, *Pneumococcus*, *Streptococcus* group A and others have also been observed.

The majority of these patients develop pneumatoceles following the pulmonary infection. The bronchopulmonary episodes appear early, even as early as the first day of life. There is usually a history of pruriginous dermatitis of early appearance, and retarded physical growth (Figure 8.3). The mode of inheritance is not yet clear, but it seems that it may be inherited as an autosomal dominant with

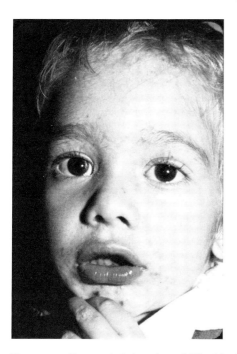

Figure 8.3. Eczematic lesions in a child with the hyper-IgE syndrome (courtesy of Dr. D. Garcia de Olarte, Universidad de Antioquia, Colombia).

variable penetrance. Some have classified this hyper-IgE syndrome as a disorder of phagocytosis, particularly chemotaxis. The latter, however, is normal in a large number of patients, and it is virtually certain that this is not the basic problem in these patients. It seems clear, however, that there are defects of the cellular immune system in these individuals, and it is not only a humoral defect. Job's syndrome, with high levels of IgE occurring in women with red hair and very fair skin, may be a variant of this hyperimmunoglobulin E syndrome, and not a separate entity.

Hypoimmunoglobulin E syndrome

These cases are still rarer than the foregoing. Very few cases, perhaps only two, have been reported with selective deficiency of IgE with chronic pulmonary disease and associated bronchiectasis.

Ataxia telangiectasia is frequently associated with deficiency of IgA and IgE, but the absence of the latter does not seem to influence the clinical manifestations of the disease, since bronchopulmonary infections are equally frequent in ataxia telangiecta￼ ￼ with or without IgE deficiency. This is contrary to what has been observed ￼n selective deficiency of IgA.

Treatment

There is no specific treatment for the IgE problems. Plasma infusions may be used if the severity of the disease makes it necessary, but this may induce the production of anti-IgE antibodies.

8.7. Subgroup deficiencies

These are very rare types of immunodeficiency in which there is absence of one or more of the subgroups of any one immunoglobulin. Generally there are no major changes in the total levels of the immunoglobulin in question.

There is also increased susceptibility to infection, similar to that observed in agammaglobulinaemia. The treatment with gammaglobulin in the cases described has been useful.

Deficiency of transcobalamin II

Transcobalamin II is a protein necessary for the intracellular transport of vitamin B12; its deficiency has been associated with pan-hypogammaglobulinaemia with normal T-cell function and a normal number of B lymphocytes. It seems that the deficiency of transcobalamin II blocks the clonal expansion and maturation of the plasma cells without affecting other functions of the immune system. The symptomatology and the levels of antibodies become normal dramatically with the administration of vitamin B12.

8.8. Defects of T cells

General considerations

T-cell defects are associated with a great variety of clinical problems. They can in general affect any organ, but there are specific types of pathology that are seen frequently. Among them there are extreme manifestations of common viral diseases, profuse mucopurulent rhinorrhoea, acute pneumonia usually due to *Neumocistis carinii* or cytomegalovirus and haematological disorders. The majority of the patients with T-cell defects have at least one of these manifestations, but there are also minor disorders in this group, not detectable by present-day methods, that will be more apparent as the techniques become more sophisticated.

Evaluation of T-cell-mediated immunity is complex. The easier methods (such as lymphocyte count and thymic shadow on thoracic X-rays) are useful only in extreme cases. Delayed hypersensitivity reactions, if positive, are good evidence of intact cellular immunity, but if they are negative, they do not necessarily indicate

Table 8.3. Total number of E rosettes per mm^3 according to age.†

Age	Number of E rosettes/mm^3
1 week to 18 months	1620–4320
18 months to 10 years	590–3090
Adults	750–3070

†After Fleisher *et al.* (1975).

an immunodeficiency. The quantitation of the number of T cells and the functional response of these cells are obviously more specific. The former is carried out by various methods, of which E rosetting is the most commonly used. The great majority of the lymphocytes that form E rosettes (more than 75% of circulating lymphocytes) are T cells. Table 8.3 shows the normal values of E rosettes per cubic millimetre at various ages. However, it is important to note that a normal number of E rosettes in a patient does not rule out a cellular immunodeficiency. In the many who have normal numbers of rosettes, functional responses of T cells should be evaluated by various methods which include proliferative response to various antigenic stimuli, ability to release soluble products, and the study of cell subpopulations.

Classification

Although there are several defects which have been defined as primary deficiencies of T cells, three of them are really important: the Di George syndrome, the nucleoside phosphorylase deficiency and cartilage-hair hypoplasia.

The Di George syndrome

This was first described in 1968, although there were several cases published before then which were not recognized as forms of this syndrome. Two forms are recognized: complete, with neonatal hypocalcaemia and thymic aplasia, and partial with neonatal tetany and thymic hypoplasia (Figure 8.4). This syndrome does not appear to be genetically determined, although there is a report of two affected sibs in the same family whose mother also had hypoparathyroidism and diminished cellular immunity, suggesting autosomal dominant inheritance. A possible genetic variant is perhaps recessive, but it causes a defect in intra-uterine growth and fetal death. The mechanism that produces the anomalies of parathyroid, thymus, aortic arch and facial structure in this entity is unknown, but its presence in some children with cytogenetic abnormalities and in other syndromes of various inheritance types make the existence of a single etiological factor unlikely.

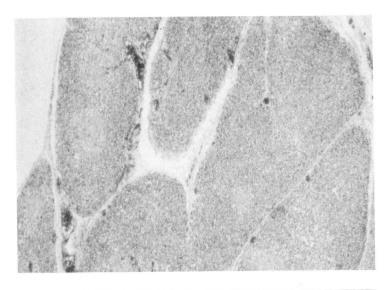

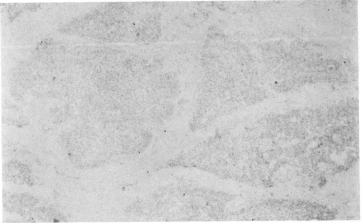

Figure 8.4. Structure of the (*a*) normal thymus by comparison with a (*b*) hypoplastic one.

Clinical manifestations

The symptomatology varies greatly according to the level of thymic hypoplasia. Severe hypocalcaemia is usually observed during the first month of life in the complete form, with low concentrations of calcium and parathyroid hormones. In these cases the diagnosis of thymic aplasia can only be confirmed at necropsy, carefully excluding an ectopic thymus. In the less severe forms of the disease it may manifest during the first year of life, with diarrhoea or chronic rhinitis, oral candidiasis or interstitial pneumonia. In laboratory studies, these patients show a diminished number of E rosettes, diminution of the lymphocyte response to various antigenic stimuli, and hypoplasia or absence of the thymus shown in thoracic X-rays.

Other anomalies have frequently been described in these patients, particularly micrognathia, low-set ears, hypertelorism, oesophageal atresia, hypothyroidism and Fallot's tetralogy.

Treatment

Evaluation of adequate treatment of the Di George syndrome is difficult since cases are known of what seems to be spontaneous recovery. However, in the more severe cases, thymic transplantation has given good results with recovery of cellular function for long periods of time. It seems that the transplanted tissue on these cases is not the sole cause of immunological reinstatement of these individuals, but that it acts upon the pre-thymic cells present in the patient helping them to differentiate into T cells.

Deficiency of nucleoside phosphorylase

This is an immunodeficiency characterized by anaemia, recurrent infections, normal B cells, depressed T-cell function and deficiency of nucleoside phosphorylase. At least 10 patients have been reported. Figure 8.5 shows schematically purine metabolism and the level of action of the nucleoside phosphorylase. The mechanism by which the deficiency of this enzyme produces cellular immunodeficiency is unknown, but it is believed that the desoxypurines may be selectively trapped by the thymus and lymphoid cells in the absence of nucleoside phosphorylase and that these produce cellular toxicity.

Clinical manifestation

The original case in which the immunodeficiency was described was a five-year-old girl with recurrent infections from four months of age and anaemia with erythroid hypoplasia. Immunological studies showed normal B-cell function, with adequate levels of immunoglobulins and normal response to immunization with various antigens. However, the study of T cells showed a diminished number of E rosettes, no response to stimulation of lymphocytes with phytohaemaglutinin *in vitro*, negative delayed hypersensitivity reaction, and persistent lymphopenia. Electrophoresis of red-cell lysates showed the absence of nucleoside phosphorylase in the patient, with unusual electrophoretic patterns in both parents, who also had levels of this enzyme at about 50% of the normal. The electrophoretic variants of this enzyme are inherited as autosomal codominants and the structural locus has been located by cellular hybridization on chromosome 14.

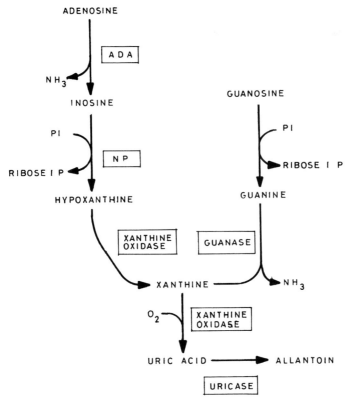

Figure 8.5. Diagram of purine metabolism showing the level of action of nucleoside phosphorylase (NP) and adenosine deaminase (ADA).

Treatment

This patient received thymosine with good initial results, but there was a sensitivity reaction and the treatment had to be stopped. It has recently been suggested that uridine may be of some use and it has also been observed that desoxycytidine inhibits cytotoxicity of the desoxypurines *in vitro* and may therefore be useful in the management of these patients.

Cartilage-hair hypoplasia

This disorder was first found in patients of the Amish religious order which is an isolated religious group, but it has also been observed in other populations. Basically, it consists of a form of dwarfism with short extremities which on X-ray appear as a metaphyseal dysostosis. Cartilage biopsy usually shows a marked hypoplasia and the hair is brittle and fair (see Figure 8.6). This triad is invariably

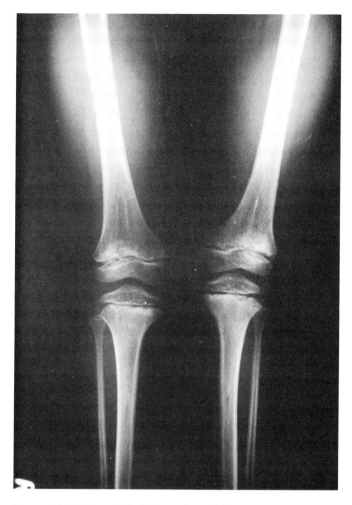

Figure 8.6. Radiographic findings in a girl with cartilage-hair hypoplasia, showing the metaphyseal ends scalloped and irregularly sclerotic (courtesy of Dr. L. Jimenez, Universidad Javeriana, Colombia).

accompanied by a defect of T cells and there are also occasionally other defects such as anaemia, malabsorption and Hirschsprung's disease. The pathogenesis of the disease is unknown, although a biochemical defect has been suspected. This entity is almost certainly inherited as an autosomal recessive with reduced penetrance. Treatment has been attempted with thymus and bone marrow transplants, the latter giving good results in one patient. Cytosine arabinoside also seems to improve the cellular response of these patients.

Severe combined immunodeficiency

General considerations

This is not a single clinical entity, but is a general heading for a series of immunodeficiencies with similar clinical manifestations but different etiologies. They have in common severity of manifestation and, as its name indicates, there is a defect both in T cells and in B cells.

Clinical manifestations

Recurrent infections from early life compromising various organs are the most frequent clinical sign. Infectious dermatitis and skin abcesses, intractable diarrhoea leading to malnutrition, chronic pneumopathies and septicaemia are common. There is no predilection for any particular micro-organism; pyogens, saprophytes, viruses, protozoa and fungi have been observed compromising the life of these patients.

Diagnosis

Leukopenia is usually observed in these patients with diminished number of T and B cells. The immunoglobulin disorders are very severe from birth, except for IgG whose deficiency only appears at about three months of life.

Subgroups of severe combined immunodeficiencies

The various defects which lead to a combined deficiency of T and B cells allow the distinction of separate subgroups. The more important — Swiss type, ADA deficiency, Nezelof's syndrome and reticular dysgenesis — are detailed below.

Severe combined immunodeficiency of Swiss type

It is believed that this type of immunodeficiency is due to an early defect in the maturation of lymphoid cells. There are two genetic forms of this disease. One is inherited as a sex-linked recessive, and the other as an autosomal recessive. There are also sporadic cases in which it is not possible to demonstrate transmission in the family, which may be due to new mutations or to recessivity.

Deficiency of adenosine deaminase (ADA)

The deficiency of ADA, which was described by pure chance in a patient with combined severe immunodeficiency, is another of the biochemical disorders associated with immunological problems and is found in some 50% of the patients with this type of immunodeficiency transmitted as an autosomal recessive. There is not a single case known of ADA deficiency without immunodeficiency.

The pathogenetic mechanism of ADA deficiency is not clear. It has already been mentioned that in nucleoside phosphorylase deficiency it is suspected that the absence of this enzyme leads to the accumulation of metabolic products with cellular toxicity. Since both enzymes are part of the same metabolic pathway, this suggestion may also be valid for the deficiency of ADA (Figure 8.5). Nevertheless, it is interesting that there are other enzymatic deficiencies known in the metabolic pathway of the purine which are not associated with immunodeficiency. This is the case in Lesch-Nyhan syndrome — in which there is a lack of hypoxanthine guanine phosphoribosyl transferase — and the three types of gout: type 1 with deficiency of the same hypoxanthine guanine phosphoribosyl transferase, type 2 with deficiency of amido transferase of phosphoribosyl pyrophosphate, and type 3 where there is increased synthesis of this same substance.

From the genetic point of view, the problem is also complex. The structural locus for ADA is on chromosome 20. It is thought that the patients with ADA deficiency and immunodeficiency are homozygous for a mutant allele at this locus and that their parents are heterozygous. However, in several patients the parents are known to have normal values of ADA. On the other hand, the existence of an inhibitor of ADA in some of these patients has been suspected. A working hypothesis at present is that a structural mutation at the ADA locus or the presence of some inhibitor leads to a deficiency of this enzyme and secondarily causes the immunodeficiency.

CLINICAL MANIFESTATION

The immunological compromise in this type of immunodeficiency is very variable and the clinical manifestations depend on it. Half of these patients have very peculiar bone defects, consisting of cupping and flaring of the anterior rib ends, alterations in the shape and articulation of the spinal transverse processes, abnormal pelvis and platyspondylia.

Different clinical managements have been applied in this immunodeficiency. Partial immunological restoration has been attained by red-cell transfusions, but thymic hormone and desoxycytidine produced no additional benefit. The latter is believed to act as a competitive substrate for the enzyme desoxycytidine kinase, which is considered responsible for the accumulation of desoxy-ATP in the T cells of these patients.

Cellular immunodeficiency with immunoglobulin (Nezelof's syndrome)

This is one of the more controversial types of immunodeficiency; it has not been possible to define it as an entity in itself, so it is usually classified as a variant of severe combined immunodeficiency. In the majority of cases there is a profound defect in the T cells but that in the B cells is very variable, with normal or even elevated levels of some immunoglobulins. The basic defect in this syndrome is still unknown. Unfortunately, ADA deficiency has not been excluded in the majority of patients. From the genetic point of view, cases have been described of X-linked and autosomal recessive inheritance in these patients.

Reticular dysgenesis

This is a severe combined deficiency of T and B cells which is accompanied by agenesis of the precursors of the granulocytes in the bone marrow. It is a particularly aggressive form of immunodeficiency in which the patients usually die during the earliest days of life. The mode of inheritance is not clear, but the affected children have no positive family histories. In theory, bone-marrow transplants should correct the defect, but a case of spontaneous recovery has also been described.

8.9. Other immunodeficiencies

Chronic mucocutaneous candidiasis

This is a difficult defect to classify since the main problem is a chronic mucocutaneous infection by *Candida* without the usual manifestations of T- and B-cell defects (see Figure 8.7). The pathogenesis is not clear and the immune defect is very variable. Generally, B-cell function is normal although some cases have been observed with selective IgA deficiency. The main defect appears to lie at the level of the T cells or the macrophages, but the theories so far proposed do not explain the specific vulnerability of these patients to *Candida albicans*.

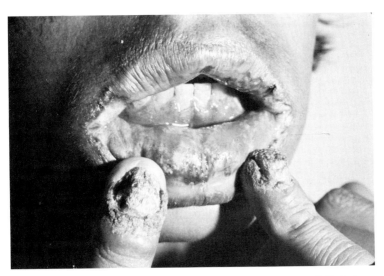

Figure 8.7. Oral and nail lesions in chronic mucocutaneous candidiasis (courtesy of Dr. D. Garcia de Olarte, Universidad de Antioquia, Colombia).

Ataxia telangiectasia

This disease is usually inherited as an autosomal recessive and is associated with recurrent pulmonary infections, cerebellar ataxia, oculocutaneous telangiectases, and anomalies of T- and B-cell functions. Not only, therefore, is the nervous system compromised, but so are the vascular, endocrine and immune systems. The immunological defects are very variable. Selective deficiency of IgA is found at high frequency and seems to be due to a defect in the terminal differentiation of the cells which produce IgA, since there are normal numbers of lymphocytes with IgA on their surface in these patients. Frequently the deficiency of IgA is associated with deficiency or low levels of IgE whose common genetic basis has already been discussed. Another interesting finding in this entity is the frequent elevation of IgM; this may also be an artefact, since a low-molecular-weight IgM has been described in this disease which diffuses more rapidly in agar, giving levels higher than the normal IgM. The cellular arm of the immune system is also altered. Total T cells may be normal or low in number; there is frequently a diminution in the delayed hypersensitivity reaction and diminution of response of lymphocytes to antigenic stimulation.

An interesting problem of this disease is the elevation of the levels of alphafoetoprotein (AFP) found in these patients which, as is well known, is a frequent finding in tumour pathology, and the incidence of cancer in ataxia telangiectasia is higher than in the general population. It has been suggested that AFP may be an immune suppressor, so these associations lead one to think that this function may be of importance in the pathogenesis of the disease.

Unpublished investigations on the immunosuppressive effect of AFP during pregnancy and in the newborn show that AFP is unlikely to have a major immunosuppressive effect, although an immunoregulatory mechanism of some sort cannot be excluded. The elevation of AFP levels in ataxia telangiectasia and in other pathologies may therefore be due to a primary development defect and not be the cause of these disorders.

Ataxia telangiectasia also shows other interesting genetic problems. The fibroblasts of these patients are abnormally sensitive to radiation *in vitro*, and chromosomal abnormalities are frequently observed in their peripheral leukocytes, which range from an increased number of chromosomal breaks to chromosomal rearrangements and translocations usually involving chromosomes 7 and 14. This cellular and chromosomal hypersensitivity has led to the suggestion that a DNA repair defect is the underlying dysfunction in these patients, although the experimental evidence remains controversial. Of particular interest to immunogeneticists is the marked incidence of abnormalities involving chromosome 14 in ataxia telangiectasia, since the genes coding for the human immunoglobulin heavy chains are on that chromosome. These patients are usually deficient in IgA and IgE, and the isotype switch goes from IgM to IgA to IgE by recombination, so it is possible that failure in the recombination and DNA repair in these patients is responsible for the deficiency. This hypothesis is supported by the recent observation, by use of a DNA probe for the C region, that these patients do indeed possess a coding sequence for that IgA region.

Wiskott-Aldrich syndrome

This is an immunodeficiency inherited as a sex-linked recessive, which compromises the T- and B-cell systems and clinically is associated with eczema, thrombocytopenia and characteristic ear infections. The central defect that causes the immunodeficiency in this syndrome is unknown. On the humoral side there is hypercatabolism of IgG and IgA, but maintaining normal levels of the former and usually increased levels of the latter, so that the synthesis of these two immunoglobulins is several times greater than normal. IgM, on the contrary, is diminished in these patients.

On the cellular side of the immune response, normal numbers of T lymphocytes have been observed with diminished or normal cellular response. A consistent finding is the failure to produce antibodies to antigens of the polysaccharide type. It has been suggested that the basic defect may be at the level of the T cells or the macrophage or that there is a dysfunction in the handling of antigens in these patients. Neither of these two suggestions can yet be eliminated. Recently, it has been suggested that there is a defect in the metabolism in the platelets in these patients which allows the detection of heterozygous carriers of this immune deficiency.

Bibliography

Altman, L., Snyderman, R. and Blaese, R., Abnormalities of chemotactic lymphokine synthesis and monocyte leukocyte chemotaxis in Wiskott-Aldrich syndrome. *J. Clin. Invest.*, 54: 486 (1974).

Ammann, A. J. and Hong, R., Selective IgA deficiency: presentation of 50 cases and a review of the literature. *Medicine*, 50: 223 (1971).

Ammann, A. J., Roth, J. and Hong, R., Recurrent sinopulmonary infection, mental retardation and combined IgA and IgE deficiency. *J. Pediat.*, 77: 802 (1970).

Bachmann, R., Studies on the serum γ A-globulin level: III. The frequency of A-γ A-globulinemia *Scand. J. Clin. Lab. Invest.*, 17: 316 (1965).

Biggar, W. D. and Good, R. A., Immunodeficiency in ataxia-telangiectasia. *Birth Defects Original Article Series*, 1: 271 (1975).

Buckley, R. H. and Becker, W. G., Abnormalities in regulation of human IgE synthesis. *Immunological Rev.*, 41: 288 (1978).

Buckley, R. H., Wray, B. B. and Belmaker, E. Z., Extreme hyperimmunoglobulinemia E and undue susceptibility to infection. *Pediatrics*, 49: 59 (1972).

Bull, D. M. and Tomasi, T. B., Deficiency of immunoglobulin A in intestinal disease. *Gastroenterology*, 54: 313 (1968).

Candy, D. C. A., Hayward, A. R., Hughes, D. T., Layward, L. and Soothill, J. F., Four families with immunodeficiency and chromosomal abnormalities. *Arch. Dis. Child.*, 54: 518 (1979).

Cooper, M. D., Lawton, A. R., Pred'homme, J. L. and Seligmann, M., Primary antibody deficiencies. *Springer Semin. Immunopathol.*, 1: 264 (1978).

Davis, E. G., Levinsky, R. J., Webster, D. R., Simmonds, H. A. and Perrett, D., Effect of red cell transfusions, thymic hormone and deoxycytidine in severe combined immunodeficiency due to adenosine deaminase deficiency. *Clin. Exp. Immunol.*, 50: 303 (1982).

Dawson, J., Hodgson, H. J. F., Pepys, M. B., Peters, T. J. and Chadwick, V. S., Immunodeficiency, malabsorption and secretory diarrhea. A new syndrome. *Am. J. Med.*, **67**: 540 (1979).

Eibl, M. M. Mannhalter, J. W., Zielinski, C. C. and Ahmad, R., Defective macrophage–T-cell interaction in common varied immunodeficiency. *Clin. Immunol. Immunopathol.*, **22**: 316 (1982).

Fleisher, T. A., Luckasen, J. R., Sabad, A., Gehrtz, R. C. and Kersey, J. H., T and B lymphocyte subpopulations in children. *Pediatrics*, **55**: 162 (1975).

Fontan, G., De la Concha, E. G., Garcia Rodriguez, M. C., Zabay, J. M., Carrasco, S., Alba, J., Pascual-Salcedo, D. and Ojeda, J. A., Severe combined immunodeficiency with disbalance and functional abnormalities in the T-lymphocyte subsets. *Clin. Immunol. Immunopathol.*, **24**: 432 (1982).

Friedmann, M., Fialkow, P. J., Davis, S. D., Ochs, H. D. and Wedgewood, R. J., Autoimmunity in the relatives of patients with immunodeficiency diseases. *Clin. Exp. Immunol.*, **28**: 375 (1977).

Giblett, E. R., Anderson, J. E., Cohen, I., Pollara, B. and Meuwissen, H. J., Adenosine-deaminase deficiency in two patients with severely impaired cellular immunity. *Lancet*, **ii**: 1067 (1972).

Giblett, E. R., Ammann, A. J., Wara, D., Sandman, R. and Diamond, L. K., Nucleoside-phosphorylase deficiency in a child with severely defective T-cell immunity and normal B-cell immunity. *Lancet*, **i**: 1010 (1975).

Goldberg, L. S., Barnett, E. V. and Fundenberg, H. H., Selective absence of IgA: a family study. *J. Lab. Clin. Med.*, **72**: 204 (1968).

Hausser, C., Virelizier, J. L., Buriot, D. and Griscelli, C., Common variable hypogammaglobulemia in children. *Am. J. Dis. Child.*, **137**: 833 (1983).

Hill, H. R., The syndrome of hyperimmunoglobulinemia E and recurrent infections. *Am. J. Dis. Child.*, **136**: 767 (1982).

Hill, H. R. and Quie, P. G., Raised serum IgE levels and defective neutrophil chemotaxis in three children with eczema and recurrent bacterial infections. *Lancet*, **i**: 183 (1974).

Hobbs, J. R., Milner, R. D. G. and Watt, P. J., Gamma M deficiency predisposing to meningococcal septicaemia. *Br. Med. J.*, **4**: 583 (1967).

Keller, R. H., Atwater, J. S., Martin, R. A. and Tomasi, T. B., Ataxia-telangiectasia, immunodeficiency and AFP: is there a relationship? In *Prevention of Neural Tube Defects. UCLA Forum in Medical Sciences*, edited by B. F. Crandall and M. A. B. Brazier. Academic Press, New York (1978).

Knudsen, B. and Dissing, J., Adenosine deaminase deficiency in a child with severe combined immunodeficiency. *Clin. Genet.*, **4**: 344 (1973).

Kwitko, A. D., Roberts-Thompson, P. J. and Shearman, D. J. C., Low molecular weight IgM in selective IgA deficiency. *Clin. Exp. Immunol.*, **50**: 198 (1982).

McKusick, V. A., Eldridge, R., Hostetler, J. A., Egeland, J. A. and Ruangwit, U., Dwarfism in the Amish. II. Cartilage-hair hypoplasia. *Bull. Johns Hopkins Hosp.*, **116**: 285 (1965).

Meuwissen, H. J., Parker, K. and Cook, B., Inborn errors of specific immunity: adenosine deaminase deficiency and purine nucleoside phosphorylase deficiency. In *Inborn Errors of Immunity and Phagocytosis*, edited by F. Guttler, J. W. T. Seakins and R. A. Harkness. MTP Press Ltd, Lancaster (1979).

Miller, J. D., Bowker, B. M., Cole, D. E. C. and Guyda, H. J., DiGeorge syndrome in monozygotic twins. *Am. J. Dis. Child.*, **137**: 438 (1983).

Pahwa, R. N., Pahwa, S. G., O'Reilly, R., Smithwick, E. M. and Good, R. A. Immunodeficiency diseases — a review. In *Inborn Errors of Immunity and Phagocytosis*, edited by F. Guttler, J. W. T. Seakins and R. A. Harkness. MTP Pres Ltd, Lancaster (1979).

Pandolfi, F., Quinti, I., Frielingsdorf, A., Goldstein, G., Businco, L. and Auti, F., Abnormalities of regulatory T-cell subpopulations in patients with primary immunoglobulin deficiencies. *Clin. Immunol. Immunopathol.*, **22**: 323 (1982).

Sussman, G. L., Rivera, V. J. and Kohler, P. F., Transition from systemic lupus erythematosus to common variable hypogammaglobulinemia. *Ann. Internal Med.*, **99**: 32 (1983).

Waldmann, T., Misiti, J., Nelson, D. L. and Kraemer, K. H., Ataxia-telangiectasia: a multisystem hereditary disease with immunodeficiency, impaired organ maturation, X-ray hypersensitivity and a high incidence of neoplasia. *Ann. Intern. Med.*, **99**: 367 (1983).

Chapter 9. Complement deficiencies and pathological associations

The factors which regulate the changes in concentration of plasma proteins are complex and little known. The concentration at a given moment of any plasma protein is determined by its rate of synthesis, its distribution and its rate of catabolism.

It has been suggested that some hormones are involved. Androgens and adrenocorticosteroids stimulate the production of C3. The concentration of C5 in the mouse is twice as high in the male as in the female, which suggests some sex-hormone effect. In our own work we have observed that the levels of C4 are higher post-menopausally as well as during pregnancy, which may be explained by an effect of gonadotropins. In fact, children receiving gonadotropins for the treatment of cryptorchidism seem to show a sharp increase of C4, but not C3 or BF after the administration of the first dose. It has also been observed that androgens stimulate the synthesis of the inhibitor of C1 in some patients with inherited angioneurotic oedema. It is clear, therefore, that there are external, non-genetic, influences on the normal levels of these proteins.

The genetic factors are however, less clear. There are very few family studies of the normal levels of these components that have evaluated the degree to which they are genetically controlled. A recent study of 50 normal families suggested that the levels of C4 are inherited more in polygenic than in classical Mendelian mode, but there is also a pronounced maternal influence. The same may perhaps apply to other components of complement.

In general it may be said that a genetic deficiency of a given component would result from a defect at one of three levels (see Figure 9.1):

1. Total absence of synthesis of one or more polypeptides which make up an active component, due to the failure of function of a structural gene or of a regulator.

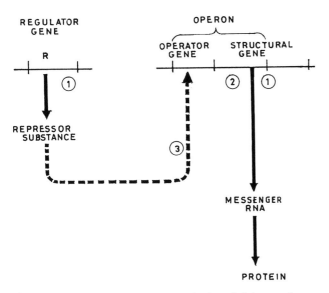

Figure 9.1. Mechanisms which may lead to deficiency of a component of complement.

2. Production of a functionally inactive component due to a defect in a structural gene.

3. Continuing synthesis of a specific inhibitor by derepression of a regulator gene.

Table 9.1. Complement deficiencies.

Deficiency	Mechanism of inheritance	Associated pathology
C1q	Autosomal recessive?	Glomerulonephritis
C1r	Autosomal recessive	SLE—arthralgias
C1s	?	SLE
C1 INH	Autosomal dominant	Hereditary angioneurotic oedema
C4	Autosomal recessive — HLA linked	Autoimmune
C2	Autosomal recessive — HLA linked	Autoimmune
C3	Autosomal recessive	Recurrent infections — nephritis
C3 INACT	Autosomal recessive?	Recurrent infections
C5	Autosomal recessive?	SLE — recurrent infections
C6	Autosomal recessive	Meningococcal meningitis — SLE
C7	Autosomal recessive?	Neisserial infections — glomerulonephritis
C6 + C7	Autosomal recessive?	Chronic meningococcaemia
C8	Autosomal recessive?	Gonococcal infections, lupus-like disease

The genes which produce deficiency in one of the components of complement are indicated as C^o or CD. Such deficiencies usually manifest as autosomal recessives, while some relatives of the patients frequently have low levels of the component (approximately half the normal values) and are therefore considered as heterozygous for the C^o gene; that is to say they have a deficient gene, C^o, and a normal one.

As has been mentioned, the genes which code for some of these components are linked to the major histocompatibility complex, and so are some of those responsible for their deficiencies. Others segregate independently of the HLA, since their loci are situated on other chromosomes. Hereditary deficiencies of most of the components of complement and of several of their inhibitors have already been described. Table 9.1 summarizes the findings.

9.1. Deficiency of C1

Deficiency of C1q

There are various reports of deficiencies or marked diminution of the levels of C1q in some patients with severe combined immunodeficiency, in hypogamma-globulinaemia, in systemic lupus erythematosus and in myeloma. In patients with hypogammaglobulinaemia it has been observed that the metabolism of C1q is influenced by the serum concentrations of IgG, which explains the low levels in these patients.

There are recent reports of two cases of C1q deficiency, who had multisystemic chronic infections. In one of them, post-mortem studies showed mesangioprolifer-ative glomerulonephritis, a frequent finding in complement deficiencies for which so far there is no clear physiopathological explanation. Family studies have been negative and have not established the mode of inheritance of this defect, nor has linkage of this deficiency with the HLA system been observed in the few cases reported.

Deficiency of C1r

There are very few cases described of selective deficiency of C1r. In two brothers, one had symptoms suggestive of lupus erythematosus and the other a history of arthralgias and skin rash. A third brother died at 12 years of age with similar symptoms. Genetic studies suggest that this defect is inherited as an autosomal recessive. No linkage has been observed of this deficiency with the major histocompatibility system.

Deficiency of C1s

Very few cases of deficiency of this subcomponent are known. In these also a pathology reminiscent of lupus erythematosus has been observed. Although it has been seen in families, the mode of inheritance is not clear.

Deficiency of the inhibitor of C1

Deficiency of the inhibitor of C1 is associated with hereditary angioneurotic oedema. The disease was first recognized in 1888, but the immunogenetic abnormality was only described in 1963. The disease frequently appears in the earliest years of life and the periodicity of its clinical manifestations differentiates it from the simple oedema of histamine origin. Physical trauma is frequently found to be associated with the episodes of oedema, but usually the triggering factor is unknown. Allergies and other types of immunological problem are not frequent in these patients.

This deficiency is transmitted as an autosomal dominant, in contrast to all the other isolated deficiencies of the complement system, which are inherited as autosomal recessives. In theory, these patients should have approximately 50% of the normal concentration of the C1 inhibitor since they are heterozygous for the abnormal gene. However, the cases studied show the levels to be only about 20% of the normal values when there is a functional protein. An attractive hypothesis to explain the whole problem envisages a mutation at the regulator locus leading to the production of a super-repressor, inibiting therefore the production of the C1 inhibitor. This super-repressor would be able to block the transcription of the two homologous structural genes, and thus explain the transmission as an autosomal dominant.

However, 15% of cases with deficiency of the C1 inhibitor present in a second form, where there is normal concentration of the protein but it is inactive. In these the mutation would be at another level, affecting an enzyme performing a function similar to the primary genetic products of the ABO blood groups. This enzyme would control therefore the addition of an auxiliary group to the molecule of the C1 inhibitor. The mutant form would lead to absence of function of the molecule, but with production of normal levels. However, it has recently been shown that the metabolism of the C1 inhibitor is inversely proportional to its concentration and this accounts for the low levels observed in heterozygous individuals. This deficiency is not linked to the HLA system.

At the triggering of the episode, the majority of patients show dermal manifestations with regions of subcutaneous oedema, more frequently in the legs and genitals. The oedema does not produce pruritus or pain, and histological examination shows dehiscence of the endothelium of the post-capillary vessels and marked vasodilatation.

The most frequent mucous manifestation is oedema of the gastrointestinal tract that presents with diarrhoea, vomiting and abdominal pain, even leading to the false diagnosis of acute abdomen. In some cases X-rays have shown appearances compatible with a diagnosis of mesenteric infarction; these images disappear with the remission of the symptoms. Laryngeal oedema is another complication which causes death in one of every five patients and develops acutely or after facial trauma. Other organs like the urogenital tract and the pleura may also be compromised and it would not be surprising if this deficiency caused sterility, as has been shown in a few published cases.

On the other hand, hereditary angioneurotic oedema has also been associated with the following pathology: systemic lupus erythematosus; scleroderma; lipodystrophy; lymphoma; dyschromatopsy.

The C1 inhibitor

The C1 inhibitor is one of the proteins governing the mechanisms of the complement system. It is an α-2 globulin with a sedimentation constant of 4.5 S and molecular weight of approximately 90 000. It is not stable at temperatures above 48°C and pH values lower than 5.5.

Its form of action is basically by stoichiometric combination with the active form of C1, but not its inactive precursor. It also combines with the complex EAcC1 EAcC1, 4b which can be inhibited by the enzyme. The C1 inhibitor does not act only upon the substrates, but may also inhibit the action of plasma calicrein, preventing the formation of bradykinins and impeding the fibrinolytic and caseinolytic actions of plasmin. How activation of C1 in cases of angioneurotic oedema is brought about is unknown, but there seems to be a relationship between the complement system, factor XII of coagulation, and kinins, which results in the liberation of C kinins, thus explaining the pathological features observed in the episodes (Figure 9.2).

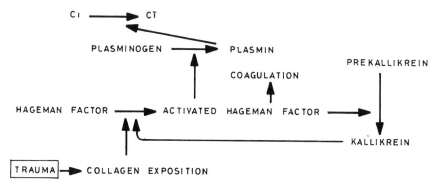

Figure 9.2. Possible triggering mechanism in angioneurotic oedema.

Treatment

Treatment of acute episodes should include fresh plasma if their severity warrants it, and in more serious cases tranxylol may be employed simultaneously. The efficiency of adrenalin is obviously dependent on the dose in which it is administered. If even with these measures laryngeal oedema is imminent, endotracheal intubation is essential.

Short-term prophylaxis is advisable if the patient is about to undergo dental or similar treatment involving anaesthesia or trauma. In these cases fresh plasma can be used, or aminocaproic acid or even androgens. It should be remembered that the administration of fresh plasma only gives inactivator for a maximum of 24 hours. Long-term treatment has been carried out with antifibrinolytics and with methyltestosterone. Among the former is tranexamic acid, *N*-methylcarbonate and aminocaproic acid. This last alone has proved to be of some value, but its secondary effects make administration and management difficult in the long term. Methyltestosterone has been used in doses of 10–20 mg per day with good results.

9.2. Deficiency of C4

This is one of the most interesting deficiencies of the complement system. Total deficiency of this component has been reported in only a few cases, associated with clinical disorders similar to lupus erythematosus. Half normal levels were observed in some of the parents suggesting recessive inheritance, linked of course to the MHC.

However, the genetic control of the levels of C4 seem to be more complicated than just the inheritance of one or two copies of an abnormal, deficient gene. The first indication in this respect came from studies in mice, where measurement of the Ss protein divided the strains into three types of animals: those with high, low and intermediate levels. It was therefore postulated that a single autosomal locus, linked to the H-2, with two alleles (*Ss high* and *Ss low*) controlled the circulating levels of this mouse equivalent of human C4. However, subdivision of these alleles was necessary because some *Ss high* alleles determined higher levels of the Ss protein than others. In the meantime the S1p protein, also coded for by a gene within the S region of the H-2, was also found to be controlled in a similar form with two alleles $S1p^a$ and $S1p^o$, the latter determining the absence of the protein.

With the initial development of techniques for C4 typing in man, a similar situation was observed, since individuals C4F (A) and C4S (B) were shown to have half the concentration of C4 of those C4SF (AB). Therefore, it seemed that either null alleles were fairly common in the general population, or there was a genuine concentration-controlling gene for C4. In fact, after the demonstration that the structural polymorphism of C4 is controlled by two HLA-linked loci and the improvement of techniques for C4 typing, a null allele was found at each of these loci at very high frequencies of up to 43% in the normal population. Moreover, the C4 locus is duplicated in some haplotypes; the C4A allotypes show considerably less (or no) activity than the C4B allotypes, and one gene product, the C4A6, is non-haemolytic when inherited with the *HLA-B17* allele but functionally active when found on an *HLA-B37* or *-B27* haplotype. It seems, therefore, that a single gene is unlikely to account for the total variation of the C4 levels, which is in fact what we have observed by applying the tools of biometrical genetics to family studies.

Although it then remains to be seen whether low levels of circulating C4 correlate with some of the C4 types, we suggested some time ago that this may be the case in spinal muscular atrophy, where we observed a high incidence of low C4 levels in the patients with a very clear family distribution, suggesting an association of this disease with null alleles at the *C4A* or *B* loci. More recently, a similar suggestion has been made for insulin-dependent diabetes mellitus, systemic lupus erythematosus, Graves' disease and chronic active hepatitis.

9.3. Deficiency of C2

This was the first deficiency to be described in the complement system and it remains the type which occurs at the greatest frequency. The first homozygous deficient individuals were found among normal people, but then patients were reported with diseases of the auto-immune type. The gene $C2Q^o$ occurs in 1–2% of the general population.

This deficiency is linked with the MHC, and particularly to the antigens HLA A10 and HLA B18. In 24 families studied, the gene $C2Q^o$ was associated with HLA B18 or HLA A10 in 21 of them. More recently, it has been observed that the determinant HLA Dw2 is also associated with the gene $C2Q^o$. From what is known of linkage equilibrium between *HLA A10, B18* and *Dw2* in normal populations it is possible that the combination *A10, B18, Dw2, $C2Q^o$* may be a superhaplotype. In fact, a recent study shows that normal HLA-Dw2 individuals have a higher incidence of low C2 and C4 levels. This was one of the first cases known in human disease in which a full haplotype of the HLA system and not a single antigenic determinant alone is involved in the development of the disease. There have been speculations about the explanation of such a well-defined association. One possibility is that all or almost all the haplotypes that have the *C2* gene derive from a single mutant gene. Another, less probable, is that the haplotype *$C2Q^o$, A10, B18, Dw2* is capable, by some unknown mechanism, of compensating for the pathological consequences of C2 deficiency, so explaining the high incidence of these genes in association with $C2Q^o$. Obviously, according to this theory, the mutant individuals for C2 with different HLA haplotypes would be at a disadvantage and would therefore be eliminated from the population.

The clinical manifestations of C2 deficiency are variable, ranging from normality to auto-immune disease. In a very few cases it has been associated with infectious problems. The most frequent auto-immune syndrome observed is a lupus-like disease. A high incidence of C2Q° is also observed in juvenile rheumatoid arthritis, rheumatoid arthritis, and systemic lupus erythematosus, occurring respectively in 3.7%, 1.4% and 5% of patients compared to 1.2% in healthy controls. These data are reliable for they come from a study where the heterozygotes were detected by low levels of the protein and the haplotype linkage disequilibrium, unlike the majority of studies in which heterozygote identification is based solely on the protein levels.

9.4. Deficiency of C3

Some nine cases of complete C3 deficiency have been described in which there have been pathological manifestations. Four of them had only recurrent infections, one with arthralgia and fever, and the other three with nephritis and pyogenic infections. These last occurred in the same family. Complement-mediated functions in these individuals were depressed to varying degrees. In one of them bacterial infection occurred without leukocytosis. In another, neutrophil functions were normal but there was a delay in the migration of the polymorphs. The other parameters of the immune system in these patients appeared normal.

This deficiency is not linked to the MHS, although there is a report of high incidence of C3-deficient heterozygotes in patients with multiple sclerosis, itself associated with HLA. This possibility has been examined by the author in 104 patients with multiple sclerosis and 134 normal controls, and the study shows that the elevated incidence of heterozygotes may be a statistical artefact due to variation in the definition of the C3 levels in heterozygotes. There is no other indication of pathological alterations in 'heterozygous' individuals for C3 levels. The incidence of this type of deficiency is unknown. We have observed a single case out of 750 individuals studied in which there was a deficiency of the C3 pro-activator, but it was not possible to study this case further since it occurred in a member of the Lambada tribe of a remote region of India.

Deficiency of C3 inactivator

Two cases of this deficiency are known. Both have had repeated infections, one by *Diplococcus pneumoniae*, *Haemophilus influenzae* and *Streptococcus beta haemolytica*; in the other by *Neisseria meningitides*. Both had a very low concentration of C3, and this was due to an increase in the catabolic rate, as well as low C5 and factor B, which are rapidly metabolized as a consequence of the deficit of the C3 inactivator. In one of these cases several relatives were found with 40–50% of the normal concentration of this protein, confirming the homozygous status of the patient.

9.5. Deficiency of other components

Deficiency of C5

Perhaps only four individuals deficient in this component have been observed, and this again is not linked with the HLA system. Two homozygous deficient individuals were found in a single Negro family. One of them had systemic lupus erythematosus and recurrent infections. His half-sister had concentrations of only 2% of the normal levels, without apparent disease but with a history of frequent infections of the respiratory tract. Among the relatives examined several were found with concentrations of C5 at approximately half normal, supporting the hypothesis of an autosomal recessive inheritance of the full deficiency.

Various other anomalies of the complement system were found in the patients. Haemolytic and bactericidal activity were diminished as well as the chemotactic function, but opsonification, phagocytosis and intracellular destruction were normal. A syndrome observed in some families, in which some of the members show a marked susceptibility to infection associated with the deficiency of the serum factor inducing phagocytosis, is probably related to C5. This is known as Leiner's disease, and has a characteristic clinical picture of eczema and infection. It has been suggested that the primary defect in this disease is a selective dysfunction of C5, since the mechanisms of phagocytosis *in vitro* improved following the administration of normal serum or C5, but it has also been observed that the C5 of these patients is antigenically and haemolytically normal.

Deficiency of C6

This is also very rare and only six cases have been published. The first occurred in an 18-year-old Negro woman with gonococcal arthritis and Raynaud's phenomenon. In eight members of her family, half-normal levels of C6 were detected, suggesting an autosomal recessive pattern of inheritance of the full deficiency. The chemotactic activity of the propositus was normal, but not the haemolytic or bactericidal activities. Other cases showed chronic or recurrent infections by *Neisseria*. This deficiency does not seem to be associated with the MHS. There is only one case reported of a deficiency of C6 associated with a deficiency of C7. This combination was observed in an English man of 70 years of age, whose children also had low levels of both components. The structural loci of these two components seem to be linked, which may explain the molecular interrelation of these two defects.

Deficiency of C7

Deficiency of this component is also inherited as an autosomal recessive. As would be expected, this deficiency is usually associated with repeated infections among which have been reported gonococcal and meningococcal etiologies. In another two individuals glomerulonephritis was found in one, and Raynaud's phenomenon in the other, but a defect of opsonification only in the latter.

Deficiency of C8

Various pathological associations have been described in this type of deficiency. There was a woman with a disseminated gonococcal infection. A second family was found with xeroderma pigmentosum and a third with a syndrome similar to systemic lupus erythematosus. This deficiency also appears to be inherited as an autosomal recessive, not linked to the MHS, although there are some contradictory results. More recently a family with a C8 molecule lacking the β chain was reported, with neisserial recurrent infections as clinical manifestations, and a case of combined C8-IgA deficiency with recurrent bacterial meningitis, but the pedigree was uninformative regarding possible linkage of these two defects.

Deficiency of β1H globulin

The β1H globulin acts together with the C3b inactivator as a modulator of the alternative pathway of activation. Two brothers have been reported with levels of this protein below 10% of the reference value. The parents were first cousins and had levels around 50% of the normal value.

General remarks on complement deficiencies

Overall, from the available data on complement deficiencies, various interesting points emerge:

1. Complement deficiencies are usually accompanied by clinical manifestations, except perhaps in the case of the C2 deficiency which has been observed in many apparently healthy individuals.

2. Deficiencies of the early-acting components tend to be found in patients suffering from diseases of auto-immune origin, particularly lupus erythematosus.

3. Deficiencies of the late-acting components are usually associated with recurrent pyogenic infections, particularly with *Neisseria*.

4. Low C2 levels and total C2 deficiency are more often found in individuals carrying certain HLA alleles, particularly *B18* and *Dw2/DR2*. It is interesting that a complement receptor deficiency (CR1) has been observed in systemic lupus erythematosus and rheumatoid arthritis, two conditions often found with a C2 defect.

5. Low C4 levels have been observed in Graves' disease associated to the *HLA-B8* allele, and in diabetes. These two diseases are known to be also associated with *HLA-DR3* determinants. It is therefore interesting that IgA deficiency is particularly associated with the same haplotype (*HLA-B8, DR3*) and that an Fc-receptor defect has recently been observed in normal as well as patients suffering from dermatitis herpetiformis carrying the same *HLA-B8, DR3* alleles. The other entity known to have low C4 levels is spinal muscular atrophy, so far only associated with HLA-B7.

9.6. Pathology associated with the structural polymorphisms of complement

As shown in Chapter 6, the majority of the components of complement are polymorphic, which means that there are two or more alleles at each locus occurring at appreciable frequencies in the general poppulation. Why, for example, are not all individuals C3S? For any polymorphism there should be, in general terms, a past or present reason for its existence, to explain the persistence of the different alleles in the population. Without some selective advantage, it is unlikely that a new mutant variant form of protein would exist at more than trace frequencies. The classic case to explain this concept is the balanced polymorphism that occurs with haemoglobin S. The homozygote for the haemoglobin *S* gene is at a disadvantage on account of haemolytic anaemia usually leading to mortality in infancy, but despite the persistent loss of *S* genes that this would cause, the gene is retained in the population by the selective advantage of the heterozygote, which is better able to resist the more severe effects of the *Plasmodium falciparum* form of malaria than is the normal AA homozygous individual. In every polymorphism therefore it is important to seek differences in biological fitness among the phenotypes, in order to explain its persistence in the population. So far the complement polymorphism most studied in this respect is that of C3, followed by that of factor B. The associations described between these polymorphisms and some pathological entities and other variation may provide the first clue.

C3 polymorphism

The first important association which is worth mentioning is that depending only on age. A study of 2078 normal individuals of both sexes in Denmark showed a continuing increase of the frequency of gene *C3F* from birth up to 55 years of age, followed by a progressive diminution up to 65 years. These changes in frequency were attributed to possible differences in biological efficiency of the variants of C3.

Table 9.2 shows some of the associations studied between the C3 phenotype and disease. The mechanisms to explain these associations are so far hypothetical. It has been suggested that in arteriosclerosis the *C3F* gene may be more active in damaging the vascular endothelium, leading to protein deposits in the arterial wall and subsequent premature development of vascular disease. The case of

Table 9.2. Some disease associations with the C3 types.

Disease	Observed change of frequency	Author
Hepatitis	Increased C3F	Farhud *et al.* (1972)
Rheumatoid arthritis (RF +)	Increased C3F	Farhud *et al.* (1972)
Coronary disease	Increased C3F	Kristensen and Petersen (1978)
Angina pectoris		
Myocardial infarction	Increased C3F	Sorensen and Dissing (1975)
Thyroid cancer	Decreased C3SF	Bernal *et al.* (1979)

thyroid cancer is also complex, but it relates only to a very small sample. There may be two explanations of these associations: either heterozygotes are less susceptible to the disease, or are more susceptible but die earlier than the homozygotes; these two alternatives have not yet been evaluated.

Polymorphism of factor B

So far this polymorphism has been described as associated with diabetes mellitus, but there are also reports of associations with glomerulonephritis and thyroid cancer. This polymorphism is linked to the HLA system, and hence these associations deserve a little more detailed examination.

Factor B and diabetes

In 1979 a group of investigators in Boston reported the first positive association of this polymorphism with diabetes mellitus. In their study of 106 patients, they found that phenotype BFF1 occurred in 22.6% of the patients and only 1.9% of healthy controls. This highly significant difference led them to suggest the existence of a genetic locus for insulin-dependent diabetes, very close to that of factor B on chromosome 6, so that the phenotype BFF1 would serve as a marker for the disease in one of every four patients. However, the experience of a group at Rochester is different. They found an incidence of only 4% of BFF1 in diabetes, and suggested that racial differences may explain the difference in the results between the two research groups.

At the same time an investigation of genetic markers and immunological variables in a group of diabetics in the north of England showed the phenotype BFF1 in only five insulin-dependent patients, in two controls, and in two individuals with other forms of diabetes. These differences were not significant, but when we took into account the age of the patients we found a higher incidence of F1, which was significant, in young patients (less than 17 years of age), as shown in Table 9.3. This finding was later confirmed by other investigators and is compatible with the concept of genetic heterogeneity in insulin-dependent diabetes. More recently, the rare band C4B4 was found in 27% of type 1 diabetes

Table 9.3. BFF1 in diabetes mellitus.

	n	FF	FS	SS	SF1	FF1
		Phenotype				
Insulin dependent	64	2	33	24	4†	1†
Non-insulin dependent	63	13	31	17	2	0
Controls	73	3	33	35	2	0

†Four of these patients were under 18 years old (*P* = 0.028).

while in only 7% of the controls in FR Germany, and hence C4 is also a marker locus for type I diabetes.

Factor B thyroid cancer and glomerulonephritis

The significant excess of heterozygous (SF) individuals at the *C3* locus in individuals with thyroid cancer has already been mentioned. It was surprising to find in the same group of patients a significant deficit of individuals of type BFS which, although it reached statistical significance, could not immediately be interpreted as a causal genetic association or otherwise, because of the size of the sample. It is therefore necessary to confirm this association. Such a double association, with an allele at two unlinked loci, may represent a more physiological than genetic association, or some interaction between the products rather than the genes.

In a similar way there was found a deficit of individuals of phenotype S in 75 patients with different forms of glomerulonephritis. The complement system has been suggested repeatedly as an important factor in the etiology and pathogenesis of this disease, and it is therefore possible that the observed differences in gene frequencies are the outcome of a real difference in their biological activity, which confers a selective advantage on heterozygous individuals over the F homozygotes. Here again there is a great need for further study before accepting this hypothesis.

C4 polymorphism

Null alleles at the *C4* loci have been found at increased frequency in systemic lupus erythematosus, but its relevance to the pathogenesis of the disease is unknown. Multiple sclerosis is significantly associated with the C4 haplotype *A4, B2*, which in normal individuals is in linkage disequilibrium with the null C2 allele ($C2^*QO$) and hence it may explain the low C2 levels observed by some investigators in this disease. In rheumatoid arthritis a rare band of the C4 pattern has been found in some of the patients. This band, called *B2,9 (Perth)* is strongly associated with HLA-B15 and HLA-DR4.

Finally the C4B2 variant has been observed in more than 50% of patients with Alzheimer's disease, while it is present in only 14% of healthy controls.

Certainly the reporting of more associations with complement allotypes is to be expected and particularly with the C4 types since this system is very polymorphic. These associations plus the identification of various alleles at different complement loci that may be interrelated in the development of a given disease, the so-called complotypes, will help towards understanding the role played by this system in the etiopathology of MHC-related diseases.

C2 polymorphism

Little information is available regarding the distribution of *C2* alleles in pathological conditions. Multiple sclerosis has been investigated, but no differences were found between patients and controls; in insulin-dependent diabetes there was again no difference in frequencies.

Deficiency of complement receptors

Besides the already-mentioned deficiency of CR1 in systemic lupus erythematosus, there are interesting genetic aspects to these receptors. It has been reported recently that there are two forms of the C3b receptor, designated F and S, individuals being either homozygous for either of them or heterozygous. Family and population studies showed this polymorphism to be inherited in an autosomal co-dominant fashion.

Similarly, another factor H-like protein, the decay-accelerating factor (DAF), has been observed to be absent from the erythrocyte membrane in a curious and so far unexplained disease: paroxysmal nocturnal haemoglobinuria.

9.7. *The significance of complement deficiencies and disease associations*

The finding of a common pattern of diseases associated to the complement deficiencies, as well as to their polymorphisms, leads us to attempt a definition of the etiological implications of the complement system in these diseases.

As regards the complement deficiencies, it is clear that some of them (i.e., the C1 inhibitor deficiency and those of late-acting components) are the cause of the clinical picture in these patients (i.e., angioneurotic oedema and recurrent infections). However, the role of a complement deficiency is less clear in an auto-immune type of disease like that observed in the deficiency of C2, C1, C4. It has been argued that these associations may merely be artefacts, since patients with symptoms of an immune disorder are more likely to be studied for their complement system; statistical examination has shown that this is probably not the case. A second possibility still considers the complement deficiency as the main cause, but not as a result of the main function of the complement system (i.e., immune haemolysis), but as a side-effect of immunoregulatory actions of the system, so far little understood. Perhaps the further study of complement receptors and the expression of complement components on the cell surface will throw some light on this point. A third possibility assigns no etiological importance to the complement deficiency, and merely suggests that it is a marker of some other gene directly involved in the expression of the disease. This theory is favoured by the fact that C2, C4 and BF are coded for by genes within the MHC, and hence the 'other gene' would be an *Ir* gene. But nothing can be said of deficiencies of components coded for by genes in other chromosomes. Besides, we already mentioned that *Ir* genes perhaps do not exist as separate entities within the genome, and hence, if it is not the deficiency in an MHC-linked complement component itself that is the cause of the disease, it will have to be ascribed to any one of the HLA determinants or possibly to several of them. The finding of whole haplotypes (supratypes) involved in certain diseases, and complement allotypes (complotypes) certainly lends weight to this possibility. The same can be said about the association of a given complement allele and a given disease. It may be, however, that there are differential immune abilities between the different alleles, which would imply the existence of a pathogenic agent that is allowed to inflict damage in the presence of certain complement alleles but not in others. Much is still to be done in this field, but certainly the complement system will turn out to be of more immunological importance than hitherto believed.

Bibliography

Agnello, V., Complement deficiency states. *Medicine*, **57**: 1 (1978).

Berkel, A. I., Loos, M., Sanal, O., Mauff, G., Gungen, Y., Ors, U., Ersoy, F. and Yegin, O., Clinical and immunological studies in a case of selective complete C1q deficiency. *Clin. Exp. Immunol.*, **38**: 52 (1979).

Bernal, J. E., Ellis, D. A. and Haigh, J., Bf in insulin-dependent diabetes mellitus. *Lancet*, ii: 961 (1979).

Bertrams, J., Baur, M. P., Gruneklee, D. and Gries, F. A., Age-related association of insulin-dependent diabetes mellitus with BfF1 haplotype. *Diabetologia*, **21**: 47 (1981).

Cream. J. J., Olaisen, B., Teisberg, P., Soler, A. V. and Thompson, R. A., Genetic basis of acquired C4 deficiency. *Clin. Genet.*, **16**: 297 (1979).

Farhud, D. D., Ananthakrishnan, R. and Walter, H., Association between C3 phenotypes and various diseases. *Humangenetik*, **17**: 57 (1972).

Fielder, A. H. L., Walport, M. J., Batchelor, J. R., Rynes, R. I., Black, C. M., Dodi, I. A. and Hughes, G. R. Y., Family study of the major histocompatibility complex in patients with systemic lupus erythematosus: importance of null alleles of C4A and C4B in determining disease susceptibility. *Br. Med. J.*, **285**: 426 (1983).

Frank, M. M., Gelfand, J. A. and Atkinson, J. P., Hereditary angioedema: the clinical syndrome and its management. *Ann. Intern. Med.*, **84**: 580 (1976).

Hauptmann, G., Tongio, M. M., Goetz, J., Mayer, S., Fauchet, R., Sobel, A., Griscel, C., Berthoux, F., Rivat, C. and Rother, U., Association of the C2-deficiency gene ($C2^*QO$) with the $C4A^*4$, $C4B^*2$ genes. *J. Immunogenet.*, **9**: 127 (1982).

Holzhaver, R. J., Van Ess, J. D. and Schwartz, R. H., Third component of complement in cystic fibrosis. *Am. J. Hum. Genet.*, **28**: 602 (1976).

Hoppe, H. H., Goedde, H. W., Agarwal, D.P., Benkmann, H. G., Hirth, L. and Jansen, W. A., A silent gene (C3 –) producing partial deficiency of the third component of human complement. *Hum. Hered.*, **28** 141 (1978).

Iida, K., Mornaghi, R. and Nussenzwelg, V., Complement receptor (CR1) deficiency in erythrocytes from patients with systemic lupus erythematosus. *J. Exp. Med.*, **155**: 1427 (1982).

Jersild, C., Rubinstein, P. and Day, N. K., The HLA system and inherited deficiencies of the complement system. *Transplant. Rev.*, **32**: 43 (1976).

Kristensen, B. and Petersen, B., Association between coronary heart disease and the *C3f*-gene in essential hypertension. *Circulation*, **58**: 622 (1978).

Leddy, J. P., Griggs, R. C., Klenperer, N. R. and Frank, M. M., Hereditary complement (C2) deficiency with dermatomyositis. *Am. J. Med.*, **58**: 83 (1975).

McLean, R. H., Peter, G., Gold, R., Guerra, L., Yunis, E. J. and Kreutzer, D. L., Familial deficiency of C5 in human: intact but deficient alternative complement pathway activity. *Clin. Immunol. Immunopathol.*, **21**: 62 (1981).

Molina, C., Brun, J., Coulet, M., Betail, G., Wahl, D. and Hartmann, L., Diagnostic and therapeutic problems associated with hereditary deficiency of the C1 esterase inhibitor. *Clin. Allergy*, **7**: 127 (1977).

O'Neill, G. J., Nerl, C. W., Kay, P. H., Christiansen, F. T., McCluskey, J. and Dawkins, R. L., Complement C4 is a marker for adult rheumatoid arthritis. *Lancet*, **24**: 214 (1982).

Pangburn, M. K., Schreiber, R. D. and Muller-Eberhard, H. J., Deficiency of an erythrocyte membrane protein with complement regulatory activity in paroxysmal nocturnal hemoglobinuria. *Proc. Natl Acad. Sci. USA*, **80**: 5430 (1983).

Pussell, B. A., Bourke, E., Nayef, M., Morris, S. and Peters, D. K., Complement deficiency and nephritis. *Lancet*, **i**: 675 (1980).

Raum, D., Alper, C. A., Stein, K. and Gabbey, K. H., Genetic marker for insulin-dependent diabetes mellitus. *Lancet*, **i**: 1201 (1979).

Rittner, C. and Bertrams, J., On the significance of C2, C4 and factor B polymorphisms in disease. *Hum. Genet.*, **56**: 235 (1981).

Schroder, R., Zander, H., Andreas, A. and Mauff, G., Multiple sclerosis: immunogenetic analysis of sib-pair double case families. II. Studies on the association of multiple sclerosis with C2, C4, BF, C3, C6 and GLO polymorphisms. *Immunobiology*, **164**: 160 (1983).

Shokeir, M. H. K., The genetics of hereditary angioedema: a hypothesis. *Clin. Genet.*, **4**: 494 (1973).

Snyderman, R., Durack, D. T., McCarty, G. A., Ward, F. E. and Meadows, L., Deficiency of the fifth component of complement in human subjects. *Am. J. Med.*, **67**: 638 (1979).

Sorensen, H. and Dissing, J., Association between *C3f* gene and atherosclerotic vascular diseases. *Hum. Hered.*, **25**: 279 (1975).

Tadesco, F., Silvani, C. M., Agelli, M., Giovanetti, A. M. and Bombardieri, S., A lupus-like syndrome in a patient with deficiency of the sixth component of complement. *Arthritis Rheum.*, **24**: 1438 (1981).

Thompson, R. A. and Winterborn, M. H., Hypocomplementaemia due to a genetic deficiency of β1H globulin. *Clin. Exp. Immunol.*, **46**: 110 (1981).

Trouillas, P. and Betuel, H., Hypocomplementaemic and normocomplementaemic multiple sclerosis. *J. Neurol. Sci.*, **32**: 425 (1977).

Vergani, D., Johnston, C., Abdullah, N. B. and Barnett, A. H., Low serum C4 concentrations: an inherited predisposition to insulin dependent diabetes? *Br. Med. J.*, **286**: 926 (1983).

Vergani, D., Wells, L., Larcher, V. F., Nasaruddin, B. A., *et al.*, Genetically determined low C4: a predisposing factor to autoimmune chronic active hepatitis. *Lancet*, **ii**: 294 (1985).

Weitkamp, L. R., Barbosa, J., Guttermsen, S. and Johnson, S., Insulin-dependent diabetes mellitus and properdin factor B. *Lancet*, **ii**: 369 (1979).

Chapter 10. Disorders of phagocytosis

At the end of the last century, Metchnicoff and Robert Koch working separately showed for the first time the phagocytic properties of leucocytes, giving substance to the theory that immunity was mediated by mechanisms principally of cellular type. The concept of humoral immunity had to wait until the development of the work of Pfeiffer and Bordet, the latter being the discoverer of what he called alexines, which today are known as the complement system.

Although the importance of the phagocyte is therefore a very old concept, disorders of their activities have only recently become known and there is much still to be learnt in this field.

10.1. The phagocytic system

The phagocytic system is composed of three types of cells, the polymorphonuclear neutrophil, the monocyte macrophages and the polymorphonuclear eosinophils. Although each of these is capable of bringing about the complete process of phagocytosis, the most important of them are the polymorphonuclear neutrophils that predominate in the circulatory stream and the bone marrow and play an important role in the eradication of pyogenic processes and certain fungal infections localized extravascularly. The phagocytic system starts, as can be seen in Figure 10.1, by the bacterial activation of three humoral systems; the complement, the kinins and the plasmin. Activation of complement leads to the production of its fragments C3a and C5a, which are the more potent chemotactic agents. They act upon the phagocyte which then passes through the vascular wall towards the inflammatory site. At the same time the bacteria are being prepared for phagocytosis by the process of opsonification, in which they are covered with specific antibodies, the Fc region of which have receptors in the membrane of the phagocyte. By means of these receptors or those of the C3b fragment also present in the membrane of the polymorphonuclear neutrophil and of the macrophage, contact is established between the bacteria and the phagocyte, which is followed

133

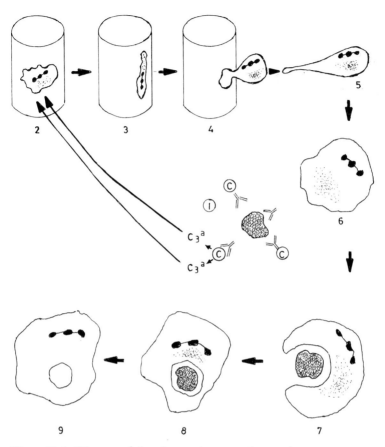

Figure 10.1. Diagram of the phagocytic process (see text).

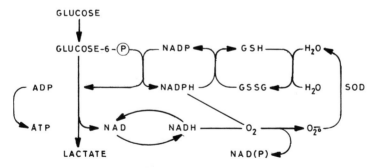

Figure 10.2. Metabolism of the phagocyte.

Table 10.1. Phagocytic defects.

(1) General defects
Neutropenia: cyclic
congenital
Lichtenstein syndrome
(2) Syndromes of phagocytic dysfunction
Humoral defects: immunodeficiencies
complement deficiencies
Defects in the response or motility of the phagocyte: Chediak-Higashi syndrome
Actin defects
(3) Defects in the metabolism of the phagocyte
Chronic granulomatous disease: X-linked
recessive
Myeloperoxidase deficiency
(4) Other defects
Systemic lupus erythematosus
Rheumatoid arthritis
Diabetes mellitus
Uraemia
Multiple myeloma
Haemolytic syndromes
Lymphomas
Chronic myeloid leukaemia
Lazy leucocyte syndrome

by invagination of the membrane of the phagocyte, the formation of a vacuole, and the internalization of the bacterium. This last process is accompanied by degranulation of the phagocyte, the liberation of hydrolytic enzymes and the peroxidase contents of the phagocytic vacuole, and marked changes in the consumption of oxygen. This leads to the formation of reduced oxygen products that actively participate in what is called the oxidative death of the bacterium (Figure 10.2). Genetically controlled defects can occur at several of these levels (Table 10.1).

10.2. The phagocytic disorders

Neutropenia is an entity arbitrarily defined as less than 1500 neutrophils per cubic millimetre. It is present in a wide spectrum of diseases such as rheumatoid arthritis, hypersplenism, and some immunodeficiencies of humoral type. There are however various interesting genetic forms of neutropenia.

What is known as cyclic neutropenia is more a cyclic haematopoiesis, in which all the blood cellular elements follow a course of regular numerical oscillation. This variation is more apparent in the polymorphonuclear neutrophils, since they have a short half-life and a long maturation period. The disease is inherited as an autosomal dominant of variable penetrance, but its aetiopathological bases are unknown. Cases have been described not only in man but also in the Collie dog;

in the latter it is always accompanied by grey hair and a defect has been observed
in the germ cell layer which may also be the case in man.

Lichtenstein's syndrome was described in 1971. It presents with recurrent
infections due to a neutropenia with selective deficiency of IgA, peripheral
osteoporosis, defects in the fusion of the posterior spinal arches, subluxation of
the C1 and C2 vertebral bodies, camptodactylia, a single palmar crease,
pulmonary cysts and a peculiar facial expression. It is believed that this defect is
inherited as an autosomal recessive.

Congenital neutropenia is a deficiency which is inherited either as a dominant
or a recessive. It must be differentiated from a rarer transient neutropenia due to
the transplacental passage of antibodies against fetal neutrophils in the babies of
mothers sensitized by the neutrophils of the fetus. The congenital form is of
variable expression, even to the point of being found in adults. The majority of
patients with neutropenia, either congenital or cyclic, have very few clinical
manifestations, due perhaps to the fact that the normal cycle of the neutrophil
is much more capable of dealing with an infectious process than is strictly
necessary. In another of these variants, the infantile form of Kostmann, inherited
as an autosomal recessive, an association has been reported with HLA B12, suggesting that there may be a gene controlling the differentiation of the neutrophil
linked with the HLA system (Chapter 14).

10.3. Syndromes of phagocytic dysfunction

Humoral disorders

As noted above, phagocytic action necessitates the generation of a series of
chemotactic agents and the availability of antibodies to coat the pathogenic agent,
preparing it for phagocytosis. It is therefore obvious that a deficiency at any one
of these levels would lead secondarily to a defect in phagocytosis; these cases have
already been discussed in the chapters dealing with complement deficiencies and
immune deficiencies.

Disorders of response or motility of the phagocyte

Chediak-Higashi syndrome

This syndrome is clinically characterized by partial oculo-cutaneous albinism,
neutropenia, recurrent pyogenic infections, giant intracellular lysosomes and an
autosomal recessive mode of inheritance. The etiopathogenesis of this syndrome
is unknown, but there are also alterations at various levels in the phagocytic
process and hence its inclusion here is arbitrary (Figures 10.3 and 10.4).

Neutrophils in the Chediak-Higashi syndrome act as if they were permanently
stimulated; they ingest particles at very high rates and liberate enzyme from their
specific granules. However, intracellular death of bacteria is very slow, due perhaps

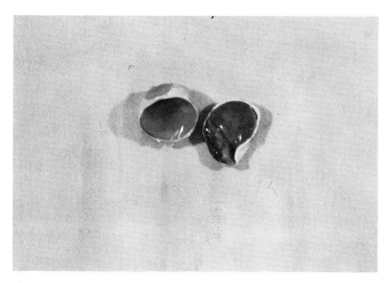

Figure 10.3. Section through the eye of a patient with the Chediak-Higashi syndrome compared to a normal eye, to show the partial albinism of this syndrome.

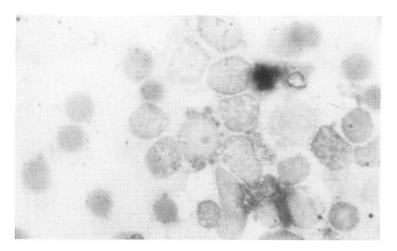

Figure 10.4. Bone marrow of the patient in Figure 10.3 (× 3000). Note the giant cytoplasmic inclusions.

to a defect in the fusion of the granules of the neutrophil and the phagosomes. There is also a defect in chemotaxis that is believed to be secondary to a defect in the deformative ability of the cell. It is therefore possible, if speculative, that the basic defect in this syndrome is a chronic activation of the phagocytic membrane which leads to all the other defects.

As a curious case, a patient is known with the Chediak-Higashi syndrome and concomitant Hodgkin's disease in which the phagocytosis tests were normal. As part of his treatment, the patient was receiving vitamin C which suggested that vitamin C might be helpful in the clinical management of these patients. Furthermore, the neutrophils of these individuals have very high levels of cyclic AMP, which can be corrected *in vivo* and *in vitro* with vitamin C. It remains to be determined whether this very simple therapy can prevent the infections and malignancies that cause death so rapidly in these children. There are also cases known of improvement *in vitro* and *in vivo* with the administration of parasympatheticomimetic agents.

The clinical course of the disease is very variable. Besides the signs already mentioned, there may be inexplicable recurrent fever, peripheral neuropathy, lymphohistiocytic proliferation in the liver, spleen and bone marrow, usually associated with intercurrent infections usually leading to death. This is what is known as the accelerated phase in the Chediak-Higashi syndrome.

Disorders of actin

It seems that a single case has been reported of a defect of actin. It occurred in a boy with repetitive infections, both gram-positive and gram-negative, in which the neutrophils did not migrate in response to chemotactic agents, and ingestion of the antigen was markedly depressed. All the cellular and humoral immune functions were normal, but investigation of the actin in cellular homogenates showed that it was not capable of developing into filaments as occurs in normal neutrophils. The findings in this patient confirm other investigators' studies *in vitro* that have shown the importance of the microfilaments of actin as a 'cytoskeleton' of the neutrophil, that allow it not only to move in response to stimulation by chemotactic agents, but also to invaginate the bacteria and form the phagosome.

Disorders of phagocytic metabolism

Chronic granulomatosis

This disease should be suspected in boys with chronic or recurrent infection by unusual organisms, especially where there is a history of death of a sib following infection. The infections are usually of a type of suppurative lymphadenitis, pneumonia or hepatic abscess, almost always accompanied by skin manifestations of eczematous type. Laboratory investigations show slight anaemia and high levels of immunoglobulins.

Although it was formerly believed that chronic granulomatous disease was a type of collagenosis of the reticulo-endothelial system, today it is known that the basic defect is phagocytic. The nuclear polymorphs of these patients ingest but are not capable of destroying catalase-positive micro-organisms, since they do not generate the products derived from oxygen that control lytic action. All the reactions associated with the metabolism of oxygen are therefore altered in the phagocytes of these patients.

Various diseases are called chronic granulomatous disease with distinct molecular and genetic problems, but similar clinical manifestations. The classic form of the disorder is transmitted as an X-linked recessive. In this there is a deficiency of the nicotinamide adenine dinucleotide oxidase (NADPH-oxidase) of the nuclear polymorph, which is the enzyme controlling the cellular respiratory process during phagocytosis. There has also been observed a variant in which there is a defect in the production of superoxide in two male patients with chronic granulomatous disease, suggesting that this variant also may be inherited as an X-linked recessive. Besides these two types, this disease has been observed in individuals deficient in glucose 6-phosphate dehydrogenase, the locus for which is also on the X chromosome.

There also exist various types of chronic granulomatous diseases with an autosomal recessive pattern of inheritance. One of these presents as a deficiency of glutathione peroxidase in the leukocytes.

In summary, Good has classified chronic granulomatosis into four types:

1. The classic sex-linked form; this is associated with the absence of the Kx antigen from leucocytes, the antigen which controls the synthesis of the precursor of the Kell blood group.

2. A form that is also present in women, but whose fathers cannot be classified by criteria for the X-linked form of the disorder.

3. That observed in lipochromic familial histiocytosis, also a recessive.

4. That produced by glucose 6-phosphate dehydrogenase deficiency.

It is obvious that at present classification is tentative and subject to considerable change.

Myeloperoxidase deficiency

The deficiency of this enzyme in the granules of the neutrophils and monocytes is inherited as an autosomal recessive. In the few documented cases a slight susceptibility to pyogenic infections has been observed, but there is a defect in the antimicrobial capacity of the phagocyte.

Various disorders of phagocytosis

Given the complexity of the phagocytic system and the great number of pharmacological agents that inhibit its response, it is to be expected that phagocytic defects occur in a wide spectrum of pathology in which neither the underlying anomaly nor the importance of the findings is clear. Abnormal responses of the neutrophils have been observed in systemic lupus erythematosus, rheumatoid arthritis, diabetes mellitus, uraemia and multiple myeloma. There is a syndrome emerging in which there is development of eczema, neutrophil dysfunction, recurrent cold staphylococcal infections, and hyperimmunoglobulinaemia E.

Phagocytic activity is also abnormal in the haemolytic syndromes, particularly in those due to haemoglobinopathies.

Other entities with phagocytic defects include lymphomas, chronic myeloid leukaemia and lymphoblastic leukaemia. The syndrome of the lazy leucocyte is another entity difficult to classify, in which there are defective chemotactic responses that do not respond to the administration of fresh plasma, which leads one to think that this may be an inherent neutrophil defect.

Bibliography

Baehner, R. L. and Boxer, L. A., Morphological and biochemical alterations of polymorphonuclear neutrophil (PMN) leukocytes from patients with inborn errors of phagocytic function: a comprehensive review. In *Inborn Errors of Immunity and Phagocytosis*, edited by F. Guttler, J. W. T. Seakins and R. A. Harkness. MTP Press Limited, Lancaster (1979).

Baehner, R. L., Disorders of leukocytes leading to recurrent infection. *Pediatr. Clin. North Am.*, **19**: 935 (1972).

Boxer, L. A., Watanabe, A. M., Rister, M., Besch, H. R., Allen, J. and Baehner, R. L., Correction of leukocyte function in Chediak-Higashi syndrome by ascorbate. *N. Engl. J. Med.*, **295**: 1041 (1976).

Briheim, G., Stendahl, O. and Claes, D., Intra and extracellular events in Luminol-dependent chemiluminescence of polymorphonuclear leukocytes. *Infect. Immun.*, **45**: 1 (1984).

Curnute, J. T. and Babior, B. M., Biological defence mechanisms. The effect of bacteria and serum on superoxide production by granulocytes. *J. Clin. Invest.*, **53**: 1662 (1974).

Hultborn, R. and Olling, S., Studies on leucocyte function by measuring respiration and nitroblue tetrazolium reduction by simplified methods. *Scand. J. Clin. Lab. Invest.*, **32**: 297 (1973).

Lichtenstein, J. R., A 'new' syndrome with neutropenia, immunoglobulin deficiency, peculiar facies and bony anomalies. *Birth Defects*, **8**: (original article series) 178 (1972).

Morley, A. A., Carew, J. P. and Baikie, A. G., Familial cyclical neutropenia. *Br. J. Haematol.*, **13**: 719 (1967).

Quie, P. G., Mills, E. L., McPhail, L. C. and Johnston, R. B., *Phagocytic Defects. Springer Semin. Immunopathol.*, **1**: 323 (1978).

Rodey, G. E., Jacob, H. S., Holmes, B., McArthur, J. R. and Good, R. A., Leucocyte G6PD levels and bactericidal activity. *Lancet*, i: 355 (1970).

Sandler, J. A., Gallin, J. I. and Vaughan, M., Effects of serotonin, carbamylcholine and ascorbic acid on leukocyte cyclic GMP and chemotaxis. *J. Cell Biol.*, **67**: 480 (1975).

Scribner, D. J., and Fahrney, D. Neutrophil receptor for IgG and complement: their roles in the attachment and ingestion phases of phagocytosis. *J. Immunol.*, **116**: 892 (1976).

Stossel, T. P., and Hartwig, J. H., Interaction of actin, myosin, and a new actin-binding protein of rabbit pulmonary macrophage. II. Role of cytoplasmic movement in phagocytosis. *J. Cell Biol.*, **68**. 602 (1976).

Stossel, T. P., Disorders of phagocytic effector cells. In *Mechanisms of Immunopathology*, edited by S. Cohen, P. A. Ward and R. T. McCuskey. John Wiley and Sons, New York (1979).

Stossel, T. P., Phagocytosis. *N. Engl. J. Med.*, **290**: 717 (1974).

Weiden, P. L., Robinett, B., Graham, T. C., Adamson, J. and Storb, R., Canine cyclic neutropenia. A stem cell defect. *J. Clin. Invest.*, **53**: 950 (1974).

Chapter 11. Associations between HLA and disease

Associations between human diseases and polymorphic systems have been mentioned repeatedly in earlier pages. Undoubtedly the HLA system is one of the most important in this respect, although the exponential growth of reported associations obscures evaluation of their impact on the knowledge of the genetics of the immune system. Before dealing with these associations in detail, it will be useful to examine a few general points.

11.1. Studies of associations between HLA and disease

For any association between a given disease and any polymorphic system such as HLA to be statistically valid, the study should comply with some essentials in its design and analysis. Selection of patients and controls should take into account race, geographical distribution, sex, age and exposure to environmental agents whenever it is suspected that these may be involved in the etiology of the disease. There are also technical problems both in the laboratory tests and their interpretation that may also bias the results. Among those that may appear from the data, linkage disequilibrium, which we have already mentioned as a normal characteristic of the HLA system, may produce false associations. An increase of the frequency of *B8*, for instance, in a given group, may be due to its linkage with *A1*, which is common in European populations. When working with the HLA system, we are dealing with multiple alleles at the same time, and therefore there is a high possibility of finding an association by pure chance, for example, in 20 or more antigens one of them may be altered in frequency at the conventionally significant level of 5% (1 in 20). This statistical artefact, which is known as the Bonferroni inequality, is solved by multiplying the value of P by the number of associations tested. This simple operation gives an idea of the statistical strength of the association, but unfortunately it may also introduce an error of a different kind, the

142

removal of a valid association (a type 2 error). Negative associations are more difficult to prove than positives. Family studies are useful, in which the absence of a given antigen in the patients, and its normal distribution in the unaffected relatives, may suggest that it has a protective effect. Unfortunately, large families with expression of all the possible genotypes required for this type of study are not numerous.

Some diseases show significant associations with more than one antigen at the same locus. Psoriasis is a good example, since it is associated with B13, Bw17 and Bw37. This type of association suggests that there is another antigenic determinant associated with the disease, and in linkage disequilibrium with the HLA antigens, in this case with B13, Bw17 and Bw37.

Relative risks

Frequently, the associations between the HLA system and a given disease are expressed in terms of a relative risk. This simply indicates the risk of developing the disease when one possesses the given antigen, relative to that for individuals without that antigen. This risk is calculated from the numbers of patients and

Table 11.1. Partial list of HLA associations.

Disorder	HLA association
Systemic lupus	B8, B15, DR2, DR3, A1
Dermatitis herpetiformis	B8, DR3
Gluten-sensitive enteropathy	B8, Dw3, DR3
Auto-immune haemolytic anaemia	B8, Dw3
Sjögren syndrome	D8, Dw3
Myasthenia gravis non thymomatosus	B8 in Europeans, B12 in Japanese
Graves' disease	B8 in Europeans, Bw35 in Japanese
Sarcoidosis	B7 in N. America Negroes
Chronic glomerulonephritis	A2
Sub-acute thyroiditis	Bw35
Juvenile diabetes	B8, A1, A2, B18, Dw3, DR3, Dw4, DR4
Multiple sclerosis	A3, B7, Dw2, DR2
Spinal muscular atrophy	B7
Ankylosing spondylitis	B27
Reiter's syndrome	B27
Reactive arthritis	B27
Rheumatoid arthritis	B27 (Levamisole toxicity), Dw4 (more severe form)
Manic-depressive disorders	A9, B17, B5, A3, B7, Bw16, B13, Bw35
Schizophrenia	A9, B5
Essential hypertension	B18, B15, B8
Amyotrophic lateral sclerosis	Bw35, A3
Hepatitis B	Bw35
Addison disease	B8, Dw3

controls who have the antigen, and those patients and controls who do not, according to the following formula:

$$\text{Relative risk (RR)} = \frac{F_p(1 - F_c)}{F_c(1 - F_p)}$$

where F_p equals the frequency of the antigen in patients, and F_c equals its frequency in controls.

The diseases which have been shown to have a significant association with the MHS can be grouped into two broad categories, malignant and non-malignant. Table 11.1 shows a partial list of these associations.

11.2. Non-malignant disorders associated with the HLA system

Defects of the endocrine system

Graves' disease is associated with B8 in European patients, while in Japanese patients it is associated with Bw35. Also associated with Bw35 is sub-acute thyroiditis, while Addison's disease is associated with B8 and Bw3.

Among the endocrine disorders, the juvenile form of diabetes mellitus, that is to say the insulin-dependent form, is one of the most interesting. It is evident that in this disease there is a heredo-familial component, but the question remains whether there really exists a locus which determines its manifestations, or if they conform more to a multiple interrelation between the genotype and the environment — the multifactorial model. The genetic mechanisms of the disease involve, among others, its association with the HLA system. In patients HLA-B8 is usually observed to be increased, as is B15, in almost every area except France, Italy, and Israel. Dw3 is increased only in Scandinavian patients, and so is B18 in French and Bw35 in Italian patients. The findings regarding HLA in diabetes may be summarized as follows.

Individuals at high risk of developing insulin-dependent diabetes mellitus are those who are HLA-A1, B8, B18, Dw3 or DR3 positive, and secondly those who are HLA-A2, B15, B40, Cw3, Dw4, or DR4 positive. On the other hand, individuals who are HLA-A3, B7 or Dw2 positive appear to be more protected. As a basis to this association with HLA and its immunological characteristics, it has been suggested that there are two forms of insulin-dependent juvenile diabetes. One is associated with HLA-B8, characterized by autoimmunity, microangiopathy, and a still closer association with the D region, and a second form associated with HLA-B15, characterized by a marked response of antibodies to exogenous insulin and a closer association with the C locus. If then there are single genes controlling the development of diabetes, there must be at least two of them linked to the HLA system.

Many other interpretations have been given to the reported associations between the HLA system and insulin-dependent diabetes mellitus, in an attempt to find a model to explain its inheritance. Dominant and recessive models have been tested but they do not agree with the observed figures for the incidence of this disease. A third model has been proposed in which the susceptibility to this disease is attributed to a single gene within the HLA system, of higher penetrance when present in the homozygous than in the heterozygous state. This is the so-called gene-dose model. However, the low frequency of homozygous DR3/DR3 and DR4/DR4 that has been observed in diabetic patients gives no support to this hypothesis.

More recently, it has been claimed that insulin-dependent diabetes mellitus is also linked to the Kidd blood group on chromosome 7. If these results are confirmed, the most likely explanation for the inheritance of this disease will, of course, be within a multifactorial frame, and hence the HLA alleles will be one of various other factors interacting in the development of this disease.

Natural selection and diabetes

These associations do not definitively clarify the genetic component in diabetes mellitus, but make one once again wonder how the disorder could have been maintained at such high frequencies when there must have been very high mortality before the use of insulin. Part of the answer perhaps lies in the observation that women with a family history of diabetes are on average more fertile and have earlier menarche. In anthropological terms, this observation implies that in paleolithic times the diet would have rarely led to a frank diabetes, but the increase in fecundity would have maintained a high gene frequency. In other words, in primitive conditions the presence of a diabetogenic genes was probably advantageous, and it is only recently that we have begun to pay the price of past adaptations.

Nervous system disorders

The association between HLA and multiple sclerosis seems well established, although not in all populations. There appears to be a mixture of autoimmunity and production of low-affinity antibodies in these patients that may explain in large part the manifestations of multiple sclerosis. The first association described with this disease was with A3 and B7, subsequently there was described a closer association with the D region since 70% of patients with this disease were found to possess the antigen Dw2. More recently, the analysis of antigens of the DR locus has shown that, as expected, DR2 is also found at a higher frequency in patients with multiple sclerosis than in controls.

The spinal muscular atrophies are a group of genetic diseases characterized by degeneration of the anterior horns of the spinal medulla and the bulbar medullary nucleii, without compromising the peripheral nerves. The group is highly heterogeneous genetically and clinically, and only in the infantile variety has an association been observed with HLA-B7.

Myasthenia gravis (non-thymomatous) is associated with B8 in Europeans, and B12 in Japanese. Its different pathological forms have not been conclusively analysed with respect to its association to the HLA system. Finally, in the group of neurological disorders, polymyositosis has been associated with B14 and probably B8, poliomyelitis with A3 in one study, although other investigations have given negative results, amyotrophic lateral sclerosis with A3 and possibly Bw35, and narcolepsy has shown a very strong association with DR2.

Gastrointestinal disease

Primary idiopathic steatorrhoea (gluten-sensitive enteropathy or coeliac disease) is associated with B8 and with Dw3, while more recently it has been observed to be associated with DR3 and DR7. A decreased frequency of B7, observed in patients from different populations, suggests some sort of protection conferred by this allele. Again here, as in diabetes, various models of inheritance have been tested without success. Three genes have nevertheless been postulated to be involved in the susceptibility to coeliac disease: one associated with DR3, another associated with DR7, and a protective effect related to B7.

Chronic active hepatitis has also been associated with B8 and Dw3. However, the antigen Bw15 has been found increased in asymptomatic carriers of hepatitis B, but not in the chronic active or chronic persistent forms of hepatitis.

Dermatological disease

The genetic component of psoriasis has been well known for a long time. A marked familial aggregation has been shown, and it has also been observed that the disease is three times more frequent in the children of psoriatics than among those with normal parents. From the immunogenetic point of view, the disease is associated with B13, Bw37, Bw17 and Dw2 when it is the common form of psoriasis vulgaris, while psoriatic arthritis is associated with B27, Bw16 and Bw37. It has been reported that 30% of the patients with psoriasis have high levels of IgE, but the significance of this elevation is unknown. In our study of 104 psoriatic patients, in which we measured levels of various immunoglobulins and some components of complement, and carried out typing for HLA-A, B and C with the object of enquiring if the elevation of IgE was related in some way to the MHS, we showed that effectively 30% of the patients had high levels of IgE, but none of the antigens studied showed an elevated incidence. The etiopathogenic significance of the high level of IgE observed in these patients has still to be established.

Dermatitis herpetiformis is associated with B8 and Dw3, which are the same antigens found at high frequency in gluten-sensitive enteropathy. The clinical relationship between these two entities is well known. Finally, pemphigus vulgaris is associated with DR4 in Jews, a very pronounced association conferring a relative risk of 31.

Rheumatic disease

In this group the best example of an association with the MHS is ankylosing spondylitis. About 90% of these patients have antigen B27, while this antigen is only found in 10% of the normal European population. This very high frequency of B27 has suggested that the antigen itself may be an important component in the pathogenesis of the disease. However, there are a number of families described in which more than one member has ankylosing spondylitis, but the transmission of the disease does not correspond to the transmission of the HLA-B27; for example, the father with ankylosing spondylitis may be B27 negative, the unaffected mother B27 positive, and a son who is B27 positive develops the disease. The many families of this type in which the disease and the antigen are not transmitted together prompt one to think more seriously of the polygenic type of inheritance, in which B27 is but one in a series of susceptibility factors.

Other entities associated with B27 are Reiter's syndrome and reactive arthritis. The latter develops in a large number of B27-positive individuals following infections by *Yersinia*, *Salmonella* or *Shigella*, or after a non-specific urethritis.

The association of HLA and rheumatoid arthritis is more heterogeneous. There is a B27-positive group in whom sacroiliitis and uveitis develop, while another group is B27 negative without sacroiliitis but with polyarthritis. In this second group there is an association with Dw4.

It has been observed that those individuals who are B27 positive are more susceptible to develop toxicity to levamisole, particularly leukopenia and agranulocytosis. Patients who are DR4 positive normally develop a more severe arthritis that requires more aggressive treatment.

The MHC also seems to influence the complications of the treatment with gold salts. Nephropathy is more frequent in DR3 individuals, while oral ulcers occur more often in those with DR2. The clinical importance of HLA typing in patients with rheumatoid arthritis is already becoming clear.

Diseases with immunopathological components

Other non-malignant diseases associated with the MHC include those in which there is an immunopathological component. Systemic lupus erythematosus was initially associated with B8 and Bw15, but more recently with DR2 and DR3. On the other hand, patients with discoid lupus and HLA-B8 appear to evolve the systemic form of the disease more often.

Haemolytic anaemia of the auto-immune type is associated with B8 and Dw3, as is Sjögren's syndrome.

Psychiatric disorders

At least two psychiatric disorders are associated with the HLA types. In manic depressive psychosis there has been described a high incidence of various antigens, among them A9 and B5, which are also associated with schizophrenia. Other associations have been reported in patients said to be schizophrenic but in whom the diagnosis is not sure, and in these B27 and Bw16 have been increased while there has been a diminution of B7 and A1.

Allergic disease

Allergic disease is perhaps an example of those disorders in which genetic susceptibility is polygenic. There may be specific genetic factors for a given allergen, presumably among the *Ir* genes. There may be other genes of the immune response not linked to the HLA, and finally there must be other genetic factors that determine more general effects such as the synthesis of immunoglobulins or other mediators of the immune response.

The associations between the HLA system and allergic disease are many and varied. In bronchial asthma an increase has been reported of antigens A1, A2, B8 and Dw2, and other studies in families have suggested the existence of a possible gene for susceptibility to asthma linked to the MHS. There are, however, various studies of atopic dermatitis, with increase of A1, A3, A9, B5, B8, B12 and Bw35. There associations are controversial since there may be allergenic heterogeneity among the patients with allergic disease.

On the other hand, attempts have been made to identify *Ir* genes related to allergies, based principally on dermal tests with natural antigens such as house dust and pollen extracts. These allergens, as is well known, may contain different antigenic determinants and are therefore not ideal for this type of study. A few investigators have used more purified allergens derived from ragweed pollen (called AgE, Ra3 and Ra5) and ryegrass pollen (usually rye 1, 2, 3 and 4). The results are controversial, but it seems that the cutaneous response to Ra5 is associated with HLA-B27. It has also been suggested that there may be two *Ir* genes which control the response to the allergens Rye-1 and Ra3, and that their responses are influenced by the genes that control the levels of IgE, since in patients with low levels of IgE, the IgE responses to Rye-1 and Ra3 are associated with the haplotypes *A1, B8* and *A2, B12*, respectively. More recently, patients with allergic rhinitis (cedar pollinosis) and their relatives have been analysed for their IgE response to the antigen and their susceptibility to the disease. The results showed that the high response to the cedar pollen antigen behaves as a recessive trait, linked to the HLA system. It was also demonstrated that non-responders had a set of suppressor T cells that completely abolished the IgE response of HLA-identical responder lymphocytes *in vitro*. This is therefore a genetic trait controlled by what we have already defined as an *Is* gene.

Finally, with respect to genetic susceptibility to allergic disorders, it is important to take account of the genetic involvement in IgE synthesis. As already mentioned in Chapter 3, a classic Mendelian pattern of inheritance has been shown for some low levels of this immunoglobulin. The normal levels seem, however, to be controlled by a multifactorial mechanism in which the genetic component is polygenic, and this indeed may be common to several of the immunoglobulins including IgE.

Communicable diseases

Pulmonary TB has been associated with Dw2, as well as tuberculoid leprosy. Rheumatic fever seems to be a special case, since the B cells of a high percentage of these patients (75%) reacted with a serum whose antibodies did not correspond to any one of the antigenic determinants known for the DR locus at that time, and the existence of a new genetic region associated with this disease was therefore suggested. A later study in Japan did however show an increase in frequency of the DR6 antigen in these patients. This DR6 is an antigen that is difficult to define, and it may indeed be the antigen associated with rheumatic fever.

On the other hand, there has been a study of the inhabitants of the mountain and lowland regions of Sardinia, who differed pronouncedly until very recently in the endemicity of malaria. The results show variation in frequencies in some of the HLA antigens between the two groups of populations, and it has therefore been suggested that these variations may be the reflection of adaptive forces related to malaria.

Pre-eclampsia

The genetic aspect of pre-eclampsia has been discussed for decades. A dominant gene has been postulated which would produce an antigen generating some materno-foetal incompatibility, but a recessive gene has also been suggested. From the immunogenetic point of view, varied and contradictory data have been reported. There is, for example, no agreement whether the production of antibodies against the HLA is increased or diminished. No antigenic determinant of the HLA has been found to be associated with this disease, although there is an apparent excess of homozygosity in pre-eclamptic women, particularly at the B locus. This has been interpreted as indicating possible maternal homozygosity for recessive genes of the immune response.

11.3. *Malignant diseases associated with the HLA system*

Curiously, malignant pathologies have not shown associations as varied or as strong with the HLA system. This is contrary to what would be expected in view of the following:

1. Leukaemia induced by virus and the susceptibility to develop mammary tumours of the viral type in the mouse are both heavily influenced by the H-2 system.
2. In the mouse there is a relation between teratocarcinoma and the H-2 system through the T complex; this complex, as we have already mentioned, controls the expression of the F9 antigen which is associated with teratocarcinoma and is structurally similar to the antigens of the K and D regions of the H-2.

For these reasons, the association found between testicular carcinoma in man and the HLA-Dw7 antigen is important, for it suggests the existence in the HLA system of a complex similar to the murine T.

At least two other malignant entities have been shown to be associated with the HLA. In Hodgkin's disease there is a general increase of A1, B18 and B15, but with low relative risks that do not exceed 2. The same occurs with acute lymphocytic leukaemia, in which there is an increase in the frequency of the antigens A2, B8 and B12, strongest for A2, but still with a low relative risk of only 1.3. In cancer of the lung, prognosis may be associated with certain HLA antigens, for patients with Aw19 or B5 have a better prognosis than those without either of these antigens.

11.4. *Genes for other diseases linked with HLA*

We have seen that there is a series of diseases which are associated with one or other antigenic determinants of the HLA system, but in none of them does its association with HLA mean that there is a gene producing the disease within the MHC. This association would imply, at most, a linkage disequilibrium between the antigenic determinant and a gene involved in the immune response that would condition, by mechanisms that remain hypothetical, the development of the disease. However, there are five disorders, the genes controlling which are situated very close the the MHS. These diseases are the adrenogenital syndrome (21 hydroxylase deficiency), haemochromatosis, spinocerebellar ataxia, hypertrophic cardiomyopathy, and possibly Paget's disease of bone.

The adrenogenital syndrome due to deficiency of 21 hydroxylase is one of the forms of adrenal hyperplasia (type 3) which is inherited as an autosomal recessive. The linkage between this gene and the HLA system is very strong, with a high lod score and very few proven recombinations. Linkage of this degree of closeness means that the HLA types can be used in many cases for prenatal diagnosis of the condition. Idiopathic haemochromatosis is also inherited as an autosomal recessive. It has recently been observed that the gene which produced normotensive hypertrophic cardiomyopathy is very probably linked with the HLA.

These linkages between a disease and the HLA system obviously do not mean that the same HLA alleles will be found in every patient. The HLA loci will be occupied by different alleles in each patient, but in a single family the linkage means that the gene for the disease will be almost always found with a specific HLA allele. A peculiar situation has been observed in the case of the cardiomyopathy, since besides the disease being linked with the HLA, the same HLA allele (*B12*) was found in the majority of the white patients, and another (*B5*) in the majority of the Negro patients. This situation is similar to that observed between the superhaplotype *A10*, *B18*, *Dw2* and *C2* deficiency, for which there may be two possible explanations: the linkage is so tight that no crossing over has occurred in any generation since the original mutation, or close linkage of the genes confers a high selective advantage. There is no evidence in favour of one or other of these hypotheses.

In the 21 hydroxylase deficiency the problem is rather interesting. A group of 39 unrelated Italians with the disease has been recently studied for HLA and complement types. The results showed a decrease of the $C4^*QO$ (null) allele and an increase of the $C4A^*4$ in the patients. Two main complotypes were observed in these patients: one associated with B14, DR1 ($C4A^*2$; B^*2; BF^*S; $C2^*C$) and another associated with Bw47 ($C4A^*QO$; B^*3; BF^*F; $C2^*C$).

Interactive effects of Gm and HLA

During the past few years it has become evident that the immune response to certain antigens and the susceptibility to some diseases is influenced by both the HLA system and the Gm allotypes of the immunoglobulins. In fact, important interactions have been observed between Gm (1,2) and HLA-B8 in chronic active hepatitis, between Gm (1,2,3; 5) and HLA-DR4 in rheumatoid arthritis, and between HLA-B8 and heterozygosity at the Gm locus in systemic lupus erythematosus. Similarly, the magnitude of the IgG antibody response to flagellin is also influenced by the Gm and HLA phenotypes. The possible mechanisms responsible for these interactions are so far unknown.

11.5. Mechanisms to explain the associations between HLA and disease

The biological significance of these associations between HLA and disease is still unknown. The suggested mechanisms are as follows:

1. The HLA antigens may cross-react with pathogenic antigens, and these antigens would therefore not be recognized as foreign and therefore not be treated as such by the immunological mechanisms of the individual.

2. The antigens of the HLA system may function as receptors or as part of the receptors of the cell surface for certain antigens.

3. These HLA antigens may be markers for other linked genes controlling the immune response of the individual, or of other genes which cause deficiency of specific proteins similar to those observed in complement deficiencies. The involvement of the HLA system in the cell-to-cell interaction and in the process of recognizing foreign antigens has been discussed already (see Chapter 4). In that context, it is expected that diseases associated with antigens at the A, B and C loci would in some way be related to cytotoxic T cells, while those associated with the DR and related loci would involve helper and suppressor T lymphocytes.

There are, however, three important conceptual difficulties in explaining the disease associations with the HLA system:

1. Although they imply a foreign antigen of some sort, it has never been identified in the majority of the diseases associated with the HLA system. In diabetes, for instance, in very few cases has a virus been isolated soon after the development of the disease (curiously enough, one of these few cases was homozygous BF*F1), and even if it were isolated it still had to be proved that the virus causes the disease.

2. There are many different diseases associated with a single HLA determinant. This is particularly the case with the *DR3* allele which seems to confer susceptibility not for a single disease but for various auto-immune disorders.

3. The involvement of the complement system suggests that some diseases associated with complement allotypes may be mediated by still another mechanism, perhaps related to the formation of immune complexes.

The available data on the biological role of the MHC in the immune system do not yet allow a clearer picture of the mechanisms involved in the disease associations with the HLA complex.

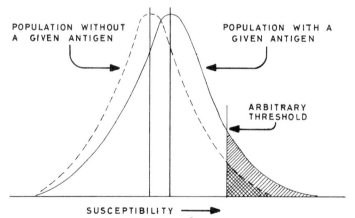

Figure 11.1. Diagram showing two populations differing in HLA type, in which the susceptibility is normally distributed and with equal variances. Shaded areas represent the proportions of individuals beyond the threshold.

11.6. Applications of HLA in daily clinical practice

After reviewing the enormous amount of material reported on associations bet-ween HLA and human disease, one wonders whether they have any defined applicability in clinical work. That is to say, would the management, diagnosis or prognosis of a patient change if we knew his HLA type. Obviously we hope that in the future HLA typing will be relevant in these areas, but in general terms it is still inapplicable in daily clinical work except in its histocompatibility aspects. This conception has a very clear genetic basis since although some of the diseases associated with HLA have a known hereditary mechanism, the great majority of them are multifactorial, which implies a threshold model of susceptibility.

There are, however, one or two specific exceptions. When considering the associations between HLA and disease, only that between ankylosing spondylitis and HLA-B27 is sufficiently strong to warrant its clinical application. If there is a patient presenting with symptoms which may be compatible with ankylosing spondylitis or some other rheumatic disorder, knowledge of his HLA-B antigens helps in making the differential diagnosis, so allowing the earlier commencement of the appropriate treatment. In very few other disorders is the association suffi-ciently strong to allow this to be done. The second useful application is where the linkage is sufficiently close for prenatal diagnosis.

The interpretation of the threshold model

Let us consider the simple case in which many factors affect the phenotype, and a variable proportion of individuals shows a complex of signs of symptoms. We may suppose that the difference in incidence denotes a difference in the distribu-tion of liability in persons with different phenotypes of the HLA. We assume that this susceptibility is normally distributed, and that the individuals may be divided into subpopulations according to whether they do or do not have a particular HLA type (Figure 11.1), which allows an estimation of the contribution of each phenotype to the total variance of this distribution curve.

We can say without equivocation that in the majority of the associations with HLA, as with the red-cell blood groups, the genetic loci involved contribute only a very variable part to this total variance in liability, and that means that they are not the only factors involved in the manifestation of the disease. Since many more unknown factors interact with the antigens of the HLA system, it is impossible to predict the clinical evolution of an individual only on the basis of his genetic make-up (i.e., his HLA type), for this can only be handled with the imprecision of the multifactorial model. These considerations, therefore, do not yet allow the study of the genetic susceptibility of an individual only on the basis of his HLA types, except when the geneticist has available full personal, family and environ-mental data that may allow him to infer the mathematical probability of develop-ing a given disease. Such cases are unfortunately rare.

A different problem is that of the diseases where the genes are linked with the HLA system (haemochromatosis, congenital adrenal hyperplasia, hypertrophic cardiomyopathy and cerebellar ataxia). In these cases, the HLA study is valuable in prenatal diagnosis or in the early detection of the disease. However, family study is routine here as well.

Bibliography

Anonymous, Genetic control of pre-eclampsia. Editorial. *Lancet*, i: 634 (1980).

Billiard, M. and Seignalet, J., Extraordinary association between HLA-DB2 and narcolepsy. *Lancet*, i: 226 (1985).

Cumming, W. J. R., Hudgson P. and Wilcox, C. B., HLA antigens in adult polymyositis. *N. Engl. J. Med.*, 24: 1365 (1978).

Darsee, J. R., Heymsfield, S. B. and Nutter, D. O., Hypertrophic cardiomyopathy and HLA linkage. *N. Engl. J. Med.*, 16: 877 (1979).

De Wolf, W. C., Lance, P. H., Einarson, M. E. and Yunis, E. J., HLA and testicular cancer. *J. Exp. Med.*, 147: 147 (1978).

De Weck, A. L., Blumenthal, M., Yunis, E. and Jeannet, M., HLA and allergy. In *HLA and Disease*, edited by J. Dausset and A. Svejgaard. Munksgaard, Copenhagen (1977).

Dick, H. M., HLA and disease: introductory review. *Br. Med. Bull.*, 34: 271 (1978).

Dupont, B., Hansen, J. A. and Whitsett, C., Association between HLA and diseases. In *Clinical Evaluation of Immune Function in Man*, edited by S. D. Litwin, C. L. Christian and G. W. Siskind. Grune & Stratton, New York, p. 97 (1976).

Gardwin, J. M., Gottdeiner, J. S., Radvany, R., Maron, B. J. and Lesch, M., HLA linkage vs association in hypertrophic cardiomyopathy. *Chest*, 81: 466 (1982).

Gattaz, W. F. and Beckmann, H., HLA antigens and schizophrenia. *Lancet*, i: 98 (1980).

Gibofsky, A., Winchester, J., Patarroyo, M., Fotino, M. and Kunkel, H. G., Disease associations of the Ia-like human alloantigens. *J. Exp. Med.*, 148: 1728 (1978).

Hillis, W. D., Hillis, A. and Blas, W. B., Associations of hepatitis B surface antigenemia with HLA locus B specificities. *N. Engl. J. Med.*, 296: 1310 (1977).

Hoffman, P. M., Robbins, D. S., Notle, M. T., Gibbs, C. J. and Gajdusek, D. C., Cellular immunity in amyotrophic lateral sclerosis and Parkinsonism-dementia. *N. Engl. J. Med.*, 299: 680 (1978).

Jersild, C. T., Fog, G. A., Hansen, M., Thomsen, M., Svejgaard, A. and Dupont, B., Histocompatibility determinants in multiple sclerosis with special reference to the clinical course. *Lancet*, ii: 1221 (1973).

Kissmeyer-Nielsen, F., Jorgensen, F. and Lamm, L. U., The HLA system in clinical medicine. *Johns Hopkins Med. J.*, 131: 385 (1972).

Kravitz, K., Skolnick, M., Cannings, C., Carmelli, D., Baty, B., Amos, A. and Johnson, A., Genetic linkage between hereditary hemochromatosis and HLA. *Am. J. Hum. Genet.*, 31: 601 (1979).

Lawley, T. J., Hall, R. P., Fauci, A. S., Katz, S. I., Hamburger, M. I. and Frank, M. M., Defective Fc-receptor functions associated with the HLA-B8/DRW3 haplotype. *N. Engl. J. Med.*, 304: 185 (1981).

Levine, B. B. and Vaz, N. M., Effect of combinations of inbred strain, antigen and antigen dose on immune responsiveness and reagin production in the mouse. A potential mouse model for immune aspects of human atopic allergy. *Int. Arch. Allergy Appl. Immunology.*, 39: 156 (1970).

Levine, B. B., Stemberg, R. H. and Fotino, M., Ragweed hay fever: genetic control and linkage to HLA-A haplotypes. *Science*, **178**: 1201 (1972).

Levine, L. S., Zachmann, M., New, M. I., Prader, A., Pollack, M. S., O'Neill, G. J., Yang, S. I., Oberfield, S. E. and Dupont, B., Genetic mapping of the 21-hydroxylase-deficiency gene within the HLA linkage group. *N. Engl. J. Med.*, **299**: 911 (1978).

Nishimura, Y. and Sasazuki, T., Suppressor T cells control the HLA-linked low responsiveness to streptococcal antigen in man. *Nature*, **302**: 67 (1983).

Noel, L. H., Descamps, B. and Jungers, P., HLA antigens in three types of glomerulonephritis. *Clin. Immunol. Immunopathol.*, **10**: 19 (1978).

O'Neill, G. J., Dupont, B., Pollack, M. S., Levine, L. S. and New, M. I., Complement C4 allotypes in congenital adrenal hyperplasia due to 21-hydroxylase deficiency: further evidence for different allelic variants at the 21-hydroxylase locus. *Clin. Immunol. Immunopathol.*, **23**: 312 (1982).

Owerbach, D., Lernmark, A., Platz, P., Ryder, L. P., Rask, L., Petersen, P. E. and Ludvigsson, J., HLA-D region β-chain DNA endonuclease fragments differ between HLA-DR identical healthy and insulin-dependent diabetic individuals. *Nature*, **303**: 815 (1983).

Patarroyo, M. E., Winchester, R. J., Vejarano, A., Gibofsky, A., Chalem, F., Zabrinskie, J. B. and Kunkel, H. G., Association of a B-cell alloantigen with susceptibility to rheumatic fever. *Nature*, **278**: 173 (1979).

Svejgaard, A., Hauge, M., Jersild, C., Plarz, P., Ryder, L. P., Neilsen, L. S. and Thomsen, M., The HLA System. *Monographs in Human Genetics*, Vol. 7. Karger, Basel (1975).

Thomson, G. and Bodmer, W., HLA haplotype associations with disease. *Tissue Antigens*, **13**: 91 (1979).

Tiilikainen, A., On the way to understanding the pathogenesis of HLA associated diseases. *Med. Biol.*, **58**: 53 (1980).

Weinberg, C. R., Dornan, T. L., Hansen, J. A., Raghu, P. K. and Palmer, J. P., HLA-related heterogeneity in seasonal patterns of diagnosis in type 1 (insulin-dependent) diabetes. *Diabetologia*, **26**: 199 (1984).

Whittingham, S., Mackay, I. R. and Mathews, J. D., HLA-Gm interactions: clinical implications. *Clin. Immunol. Allergy*, **4**: (3) 623 (1984).

Chapter 12. Blood groups and disease

When the associations between different blood groups and disease were first sought, it was expected that these would occur in relation to the infectious diseases, since the antigens of some of these organisms mimicked the molecular constitution of the blood groups. About 1960, a hypothesis was put forward in these terms to explain the world variation found in the blood groups. This hypothesis was based on historical studies of the statistics of plague, variola and cholera, in relation to the distribution of blood groups, and the discovery of antigens similar to those of the blood groups on the surface of some infectious agents. However, this hypothesis has been severely criticized, although it does not invalidate the associations observed between blood groups and some diseases. Interest in the blood groups as etiopathogenic factors has diminished in the past few years, but their value in the assignation of genes to specific chromosomes has increased. The result of all these studies is an interesting series of observations which are the subject of this chapter.

The association of blood groups as selective factors

Various chronic diseases are associated with one or other blood group. These associations are of low selective effect, since they involve disorders that are either very rare or that appear after the individual's reproductive period has come to an end. One of the most important associations, between duodenal ulcer and blood group type O, may have a more important selective effect since this disease may cause death during the reproductive period and would therefore lead to a reduction in the Darwinian fitness of individuals of type O. The calculation has been based on the incidence of death from duodenal ulcer at various ages, and taking into account age-specific fertility in the general population. From these data, it has been seen that individuals of type O have a Darwinian fitness reduced only by 0.01% by comparison with those of other blood groups. It is therefore clear that the selective effect of these associations, as with tumoral pathology, diabetes and rheumatic cardiopathy, is very low.

On the other hand, there have not been many studies of associations of diseases of infectious type. Due to the severity and world prevalence of this type of pathology, these associations may eventually be found to be of much greater selective significance than other types of pathology; a point which is still in debate, since these associations have not yet been established.

12.1. Malignant diseases associated with blood groups

Table 12.1 gives a partial list of the malignant entities which show some association with the blood groups. In general, these associations are with group A, but present quite low relative risks, between 1 and 1.4.

The first association reported with blood groups was specifically cancer of the stomach and blood group A, at the beginning of the 1950s. However, this type of tumour is also associated with group B, but to a lesser degree, and so are the carcinomas of the salivary glands and liver.

Oesophageal carcinoma is a special case, since it has a more marked association with group B, established in more than 2500 cases. It seems that the cancer of the salivary glands and of the stomach are both associated with the blood groups

Table 12.1. Neoplasias and blood groups.

Neoplasia	Association of blood group with neoplasia			Relative risk A/O	Relative risk B/O	Cases (no.)
	A	B	O			
Lip	+	−	−			
Salivary gland	+ +	+	−			
Oesophagus	+	+	−	1.10	1.29	2705
Stomach	+	+	−	1.21	1.04	6300
Large intestine	+	−	−	1.08	0.99	
Liver	+	+	−			
Larynx	−	−	−			
Lung	−	−	−	1.055	—	
Skin	−	−	+			
Mammary gland	+	−	−	1.06	—	12 000
Uterine cervix	+	−	−	1.09		
Uterus	+	−	−	1.16		
Ovary	+	−		1.23		
Vulva	+	−		1.39		
Hodgkin	−	−	+			1000
Sarcomas	−	+	−	—	1.52	216
Benign:						
Salivary gland	+	+	−	1.56		

Data taken from Mourant *et al.* (1978).

by the fact that the secretion of these glands contains, in the case of secretors, a considerable concentration of the antigens characteristic of the ABO blood group of the individual. Associations of blood group O occur in only two types of pathology: skin cancers and Hodgkin's disease. It is interesting to remember that Hodgkin's disease is one of the few neoplasias associated with HLA, and it is considered possible that this entity may be due, at least in part, to a viral infection.

Lung cancer

The great majority of the lung cancers included in the study of blood groups are classified simply as 'cancer of the lung', but undoubtedly the majority of them must be bronchogenic cancers. In the few cases described as bronchogenic cancer there is low association with group A, with a relative risk (A/O) of only 1.07. There is, however, a genetic system possibly associated with the development of lung cancer: the polymorphism of the inducibility of aryl hydrocarbon hydroxylase (AHH). This AHH is a microsomal oxidase involved in the metabolism of polycyclic carcinogens, that increases its activity when a substrate, such as 3-methylcholanthrene, is given. This increase in activity can be measured in lymphocyte cultures and classified as low, intermediate or high.

In the white North American population it has been observed that this inducibility is trimodal, with frequencies that conform to those expected in Hardy-Weinberg equilibrium, and hence the two alleles AHH^a and AHH^b have been postulated, confirming low and high inducibility, respectively. This explanation derived from the observation that in a small group of patients with pulmonary carcinoma there was an excess of heterozygotes AHH^a/AHH^b and a marked deficit of AHH^a homozygotes, which is in itself evidence of the existence of a selective process. These studies have been criticized on methodological grounds, but this does not exclude the possibility that this genetic system may have a pronounced influence in the development of lung cancer.

Cancer of the breast

The associations of cancer of the breast have been examined in more than 12 000 patients, and these show a significant association of the disease with group A, with a relative incidence of A/O of approximately 1.06. However, the phenotype ss of the MNSs blood-group system seems to be associated more markedly with this tumour, with a relative risk ss/SS + Ss of 1.69.

Other tumours

In general, all tumour pathology of the female genito-urinary system is also associated with group A, cancer of the vulva showing the highest risk. Ovarian and uterine tumours, besides their association with group A, appear to be associated with secretor status. Among benign neoplasms, those of the salivary glands are associated with A and B, as well as those of the uterus and ovaries.

Antigenicity of the neoplasias

The association of blood groups with the pathology of neoplastic type, and particularly with carcinoma of the stomach, has led to numerous studies of the antigenicity of neoplastic tissues. It is possible that tumoral tissue has a substance similar to blood group A, as a result of an incomplete biosynthesis of the blood groups in those tissues. It has been suggested that these antigens would be concealed from the immune system, but become accessible to it during an auto-immune or tumoral process. A type A person, therefore, who is unable to develop anti-A antibodies, would have a greater likelihood of developing a tumour. This would also explain the various associations of blood groups with pathology of auto-immune type.

12.2. Non-malignant diseases associated with blood groups

Infectious disease

Table 12.2 summarizes some of the data on the associations between blood groups and infectious diseases. As can be seen, in this group of diseases there is a marked tendency for association with groups A and O.

Table 12.2. Infectious diseases and blood groups.

Infectious diseases	Association of blood group with infectious disease			
	A	B	O	Other
Bacterial				
Typhus	–	–	+	
Diphtheria	–	–	–	
Streptococcal				
Scarlatina	+	–	–	
Post.Streptococcus A	–	–	–	Def. ABH secretor
Staphylococcus	–	–	+	
Pulmonary TB	–	–	+	
Other TB	+	–	–	
Tuberculoid leprosy	–	–	+	
Other leprosy	+	–	–	
Syphilis	+	–	–	
Viral				
Poliomyelitis	+	+	–	
Protozoal				
Malaria	+	–	–	Duffy

Data taken from Mourant *et al.* (1978).

Bacterial infections

Infections by haemolytic *Streptococcus* show a dual pattern of association. On the one hand, patients with scarlet fever have a low frequency of group A, while individuals susceptible to the disease as shown by the Dick test are frequently group A. On the other hand, the carriers of haemolytic *Streptococcus* type A have a low incidence of secretors.

Typhoid fever is slightly associated with group O, as are staphylococcal infections.

The associations of tuberculosis have not been clearly defined. In general there is no association with the blood groups, but when the patients are classified according to the site of infection there is found to be an increase of group O in pulmonary tuberculosis and an increase of A in the other forms. In leprosy a similar pattern is observed, since the tuberculoid form is associated with group O while the other forms, particularly the non-lepromatous, are associated with group A. Syphilis is also seen more frequently in group A individuals, and in those who receive treatment the Wasserman reaction is positive for a longer period in individuals of types A and B than in those of type O.

Viral infections

Considering together all viral infections, the associations with the blood groups are very weak, with relative risks A/O and B/O of only 0.94 and 0.96 respectively.

Protozoal infections

Malaria is a good example of a pathologic process in which susceptibility is associated with various genetic systems.

As regards the blood groups, it seems that there is an excess of individuals of type A in malarial patients, although it appears that the mosquitos possibly bite more individuals of types O and B than of type A. Taking into account all these data, it has been suggested that malaria did not exist in the New World before its discovery by Europeans, and that blood group B confers a protective advantage against it over the other blood groups which may partly explain the high incidence of this disease in some European and Asiatic areas. These points remain to be confirmed. A very important association has been reported between malaria and the Duffy blood group. Using a plasmodium which is not a human parasite, *Plasmodium knowlesi*, it has been demonstrated that the site of adherence and entrance of the parasite to the human red cell are the antigens Fy^a and Fy^b, and that the plasmodium never enters cells which are Fy^{a-b-}. This would explain the high resistance of Africans to *Plasmodium vivax*, since the majority of them are Fy^{a-b-}. The genetic importance of other factors also involved in susceptibility to malaria is so marked that it is worth mentioning. Three of them are thalassaemia, haemoglobin S, and deficiency of glucose 6-phosphate dehydrogenase. It is well known that the diseases known as thalassemia major and minor represent the homozygous and heterozygous forms of the same disorder. In 1949 Haldane suggested that the explanation of the high frequency of this disorder would be found to lie in the special resistance to malaria that some of its forms confer. Indeed, population studies tend to confirm the hypothesis that those heterozygous for the thalassaemic trait are more resistant to malaria by *Plasmodium falciparum* although there is no direct experimental evidence to prove it.

The same problem was presented in the study of sickle cell anaemia. In 1954 it was shown statistically that haemoglobin *AS* heterozygotes are more resistant to malaria by *P. falciparum* than Hb^a homozygotes. This is one of the few well-documented cases of a balanced polymorphism. Deficiency of glucose 6-phosphate dehydrogenase also confers resistance to malaria. It is difficult to explain by a single genetic process the balance among all these mechanisms. In the case of Africa, Mourant suggests that the resistance to *P. vivax* developed by natural selection through the Duffy blood groups until it was so successful that this parasite disappeared. It was replaced by *P. falciparum* for which there was no resistance at that time. When the gene for haemoglobin S appeared, the way was open for it to spread by natural selection, although the price to be paid was the loss of the homozygotes each generation.

Haematological disorders

Very few defects of the haematopoietic system are associated with the blood groups. Among them, pernicious anaemia is found associated with groups A and B, while other forms of anaemia show a pronounced deficiency of the former. Idiopathic thrombocytopenic purpura and tropical eosinophilia show similarly an excess of groups A and B.

Thrombotic diseases are of interest, since deficiency of blood group type O has been observed in women with thrombo-embolism following the use of oral contraceptives. However, myocardial infarction shows a significant excess of group A, more marked in young adults. In general, the haemorrhagic diseases are associated with group O. Such is the case with patients who have duodenal and gastric ulcer, in whom the frequency of group O is higher in those who bleed, as is the case with pulmonary tuberculosis.

Disorders of the central nervous system

Several of these diseases show pronounced association with the blood groups. Huntington's chorea, an autosomal dominant inherited disorder, is associated with groups A and B. Multiple sclerosis shows an increase in individuals of group O, and a possible excess of *cde* homozygotes in the rhesus system, which has led to the suggestion that rhesus negative O individuals are intrinsically more susceptible to multiple sclerosis development, and those observations are supported by the high frequency of group O individuals and of multiple sclerosis in the Orkney and Shetland islands to the north of Scotland. Recently, it has been reported that the proportion of persons with the intestinal variety of alkaline phosphatase in the serum is reduced in patients with multiple sclerosis, and this reduction is more pronounced in individuals of type O. This alkaline phosphatase appears principally in the serum of O and A secretor individuals, and the frequency of non-secretors is very high in the Orkney islands. The full implications are still to be evaluated, but the results suggest that further studies of intestinal factors in multiple sclerosis would be useful.

Disorders of connective tissue

Rheumatoid arthritis shows two types of association. On the one hand the frequencies of groups A and B, but particularly of the former, are diminished amongst these patients. On the other, the frequency of rhesus-positive individuals is slightly increased. Lupus erythematosus and psoriasis show an increase of group O.

Metabolic disease

There are many studies of associations between the blood groups and diabetes mellitus, which are difficult to evaluate since the disease is highly heterogeneous. In general it may be said that this disease is associated with group A, with a relative incidence of 1.07. However, it seems that this association with group A is influenced by sex, since the risk is higher in men than in women. Differences have also been observed among the age groups in various studies. In this case, the frequency of group A is diminished in juvenile diabetics but increases with age until an excess of group A is shown in adult diabetics. No explanation is as yet available for these results.

12.3. Significance of the associations between blood groups and disease

In the previous chapter we saw how the associations between the HLA system and human diseases should be interpreted as one more of the etiopathogenic factors in a given case, and that the HLA system contributes in a variable form to the expression of each one of these diseases. This concept is equally applicable to the blood groups, which contribute at a still lower degree to the development of a given disease. It has been calculated, for example, that in duodenal ulcer the *ABO* locus contributes only 1% of the total variance in the susceptibility to develop an ulcer, and that secretor status contributes 1% more. These associations with blood groups alone do not, therefore, imply any great genetic component in the associated diseases. Very little can be said of the genetic importance of these associations as long as we remain ignorant of the mechanisms by which the chromosomal segments which carry the blood group loci are associated with differences in liability to these disorders in various organs.

12.4. *Haemolytic disease of the newborn*

It is well known that during pregnancy varying quantities of foetal blood cross the placenta into the maternal circulation, particularly during the last months. This passage of blood may be sufficient to cause the mother to make antibodies against the foetal antigenic determinants. However, sensitization of the mother is much more important by the transfer of foetal blood during parturition; in subsequent pregnancies, these antibodies may cross the placenta and destroy the foetal red cells, thus producing haemolytic disease of the newborn (Figure 12.1).

From the clinical point of view the formation of antibodies against the rhesus system is the most common cause of haemolytic disease. We have already seen that the inheritance of the rhesus system is determined by a series of alleles. The most important of these is that which determines the presence of antigen D, which in routine tests identifies the blood group as Rh$^+$. The clinical problem of sensitization to Rh is then present when a Rh$^-$ mother is stimulated to produce antibodies anti-D during pregnancy or delivery, or in general by any transfusion of Rh$^+$ blood. Obviously the other blood groups may also produce haemolysis in the newborn, and in fact ABO sensitization is more frequent during pregnancy but leads less often to serious problems in the neonatal period.

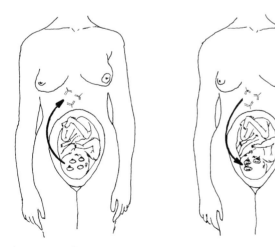

Figure 12.1. Haemolytic disease of the newborn and rhesus blood groups. A Rh$^+$ product immunizes a Rh$^-$ mother against Rh antigens. If in a later pregnancy the foetus is Rh$^+$ it will receive anti-Rh antibodies from its mother, causing haemolytic disease of the newborn.

In general, haemolytic disease of the newborn occurs in approximately 5 % of live births in Europeans. By an unknown mechanism, the incidence of maternal immunization against Rh diminishes when foetus and mother are ABO incompatible; it is thought, at least in the case of a product A Rh$^+$ from a mother O Rh$^-$, that the foetal cells may be haemolysed in the maternal circulation and the resulting debris removed in the maternal liver.

Clinical aspects

The most frequent symptomatology in haemolytic disease of the newborn is related to anaemia and icterus, which usually appears during the first day of life. This icterus may increase to levels such that it crosses the blood–brain barrier, causing damage to the central nervous system.

For many years, the treatment of haemolytic disease of the newborn was directed towards combatting the anaemia. Later, it was observed that the chief danger to these children lay in the prolonged exposure to high concentrations of bilirubin, and therefore complete exchange transfusion with Rh$^-$ blood was established as a method of choice. The treatment was extended in order to protect the foetus from other risks. These methods include premature delivery according to the history of the mother, titration of antibodies, analysis of amniotic fluid, and intrauterine foetal transfusion, in which compatible blood is injected into the abdominal cavity of the foetus. The clinical management can therefore be outlined as follows:

THE MOTHER
Maternal immunization can and should be detected during pregnancy, although there is no really safe test to establish ABO-incompatibility. When antibodies to a particular blood group are found in the maternal serum, the blood type of the father of the foetus should be determined. If the father is negative for this blood group, there is no risk in the pregnancy. If he is a heterozygote, the foetus has a 50% chance of developing a haemolytic disease (Table 12.3). If besides this the antibody titres increase, or there is a history of an affected child, an amniocentesis should be carried out in order to determine the concentration of biliary pigments.

A very high percentage of Rh$^-$ women who have a Rh$^+$ child never develop anti-D antibodies. However, all of them should be treated to prevent isoimmu-

Table 12.3. Risk of developing haemolytic disease.

Mother Rh	Father Rh$^+$	Offspring
dd genotype	*DD* genotype	All *Dd*; high risk
dd genotype	*Dd* genotype	50% *dd*, no risk
		50% *Dd*, high risk

nization since it is impossible to predict which ones will do so. This prevention is carried out by giving anti-D immunoglobulin in the first 72 hours after delivery or abortion. This treatment has recently been extended, and antibodies are given in the 28th to 34th week of pregnancy.

THE PRODUCT
Cord blood should be examined for the blood group and a direct Coombs' test carried out. If positive, this may necessitate a complete exchange transfusion although some cases may improve with phototherapy. The decision is based on clinical impression and the levels of bilirubins.

Adaptive value of haemolytic disease

Haemolytic disease of the newborn clearly represents a form of natural selection which acts against the Rh system. This natural selection is unusual, first, because it acts against the heterozygotes, and secondly because it is a function not only of the genotype of the individual but also of his mother.

Selection against heterozygotes is rather curious, since it can never lead to a situation of balanced polymorphism, but tends to eliminate the less frequent gene. For example, if a population has 40 Rh^- genes and 60 Rh^+ genes, the elimination of one heterozygote would change the ratio 40 : 60 to 39 : 59, and the elimination of another heterozygote to 38 : 58, and this would continue until the elimination of all Rh^- individuals would result in only Rh^+ individuals left. Although this example grossly simplifies the real situation, it can nevertheless be said that selection against heterozygotes would always eventually lead to the elimination of the least frequent allele in the population. However, European populations have a high frequency of the Rh^- gene, so there must be other factors which maintain this polymorphism, factors which are as yet unknown. It has been suggested, for instance, that Rh^- women tend to compensate with more children than Rh^+ women, but this would not altogether explain the problem. The recent introduction of therapeutic measures and the diminution in family size can only reduce the strength of the selection against the heterozygote.

Bibliography

Aird, I., Bentall, H. H. and Roberts, J. A. F., A relationship between cancer of the stomach and the ABO blood groups. *Br. Med. J.*, **1**: 799 (1953).
Bodmer, W. F. and Cavalli-Sforza, L. L., *Genetics, Evolution and Man*. W. H. Freeman, San Francisco (1976).
Clarke, C. A., Blood groups and disease. *Prog. Med. Genet.*, **1**: 81 (1961).
Edwards. J. H., The meaning of the associations between blood groups and disease. *Ann. Hum. Genet.*, **29**: 77 (1965).
Eklund, J., Prevention of Rh immunization in Finland. *Acta Paediatr. Scand.*, (Suppl.) 274 (1978).

Emery, A. E. H., Anand, R., Danford, N., Duncan, W. and Paton, L., Aryl hydrocarbon hydroxylase inducibility in patients with cancer. *Lancet*, i: 470 (1978).

Gershowitz, H. and Neel, J. V., The blood groups and secretor types in five potentially fatal diseases of Caucasian children. *Acta Genet. Statist. Med. (Basel)*, **15**: 261 (1965).

MacDonald, J. L., Roberts, D. F., Shaw, D. A. and Saunders, M., Blood groups and other polymorphisms in multiple sclerosis. *J. Med. Genet.*, **13**: 30 (1976).

Miller, L. H., Mason, S. V. and Drorak, J. A., Erythrocyte receptors of *Plasmodium knowlesi* malaria: Duffy blood groups determinants. *Science*, **189**: 561 (1975).

Miller, L. H., Mason, S. V., Clyde, D. F. and McGinnis, M. H., The resistance factor to *Plasmodium vivax* in blacks: the Duffy blood group genotype, FyFy. *New. Eng. J. Med.*, **295**: 302 (1976).

Mourant, A. E., Kopec, A. C. and Domaniewska-Sobczac, K., *The Distribution of the Human Blood Groups and Other Polymorphisms*, 2nd edn. Oxford University Press, Oxford (1976).

Mourant, A. E., Kopec, A. C. and Domaniewska-Sobczak, K., *Blood Groups and Disease*. Oxford University Press, Oxford (1978).

Papiha, S. S. and Roberts, D. F., Serum alkaline phosphatase in patients with multiple sclerosis. *Clin. Genet.*, 7: 88 (1975).

Vogel, F., ABO blood groups and disease. *Am. J. Hum. Genet.*, **22**: 464 (1970).

Woolf, B., On estimating the relation between blood groups and disease. *Ann. Hum. Genet.*, **19**: 251 (1955).

Chapter 13. Tissue transplantation

Although organ transplantation is not a new procedure in medicine, the immune mechanisms that have delayed its routine use have only recently been discovered. Before describing the present state of knowledge of these mechanisms, it is convenient to establish a conceptual framework for the exposition of the topic.

To perform a transplant is in a way similar to placing a piece in a jigsaw puzzle. The greater the similarity of the piece to those that surround it, the greater the possibility that it is correctly placed. In jigsaw puzzles there are features which help in the identification of the pieces: colours, shapes, etc. In the transplant these characteristics are immunological, and in general genetically determined: the HLA system, the blood groups, and so on.

The central problem, common to both jigsaw puzzles and transplants, is to find the piece that will fit, that has the same characteristics as those of its surroundings. In clinical practice this situation is only presented in the few cases of transplant between identical twins who possess the same determinants for the HLA system, do not react against each other in the mixed-lymphocyte reaction, and must be identical for all other characteristics, as yet unknown, which are important to the fate of the transplant. When an identical twin is not available, the family of the recipient is studied in order to establish the HLA type of the recipient and those of his relatives. Simple probability laws show that 25% of the sibs within a family are identical in HLA, 50% share a haplotype, and 25% are totally different in HLA. Also within the family it is generally accepted that those identical for antigens HLA-A and B are also identical for those of group D, or at least have a greater possibility of being so since these antigens are inherited *en bloc* as haplotypes.

Where there is no available donor among the patient's relatives one seeks a third type of donor: not related, in some cases alive but more frequently a cadaver. In this situation one would aim to find a donor identical for all the known systems (all the antigens of the HLA system, serological lymphocytic and others which induce the production of antibodies). This is unlikely, so one seeks a donor as similar as possible to the recipient on the principle that in general the greater their similarity, the greater the possibility of transplantation success. That is why, in many of the schemes in which volunteers promise to donate an organ after death, they may be asked to have their blood types, including the HLA, placed on record.

Clinical treatment

Clinical management of transplant patients includes essentially three aspects: obtaining an adequate level of immunosuppression, monitoring of the process of acceptance or rejection, and management of the complications. Frequently this means that serious decisions have to be taken at a critical time. For instance, to stop immunosuppression in cases of infections, although this may lead to the rejection of the transplant; to decide if a series of clinical manifestations are due to rejection or some other type of complication; to remove the transplant; these are a few of the many critical problems that may present.

With these criteria clarified, we may now consider the material.

13.1. Renal transplantation

General concepts

Of all types of transplants, that of the kidney is one of those most frequently done. The results obtained are good and improve day by day. The experience in the UK and Ireland, for example, shows that patient survival at one year ranges from 82% to 98% and graft survival at the same time from 54% to 82%.

Patient selection

In general, any patient without renal function and irreversible damage to the renal parenchyme is a candidate for a transplant, provided that he has no serious defect in other organs, and is between 5 and 55 years old.

The HLA system

As already mentioned, the ideal situation is to find a donor within the family of the patient with the greatest possible similarity in the antigens of the HLA system. If such a relative cannot be found, transplantation of cadaveric material is indicated, although it presents a serious problem still in debate: the importance of HLA compatibility between donor and recipient. Compatibility at loci HLA-A, B and C does not in itself guarantee the success of the transplant, nor on the other hand its failure. The effects of the HLA-A and B loci have been recently analysed in 700 transplants of cadaveric material carried out in the USA, where it was found that compatibility for the HLA-A locus results in a better survival than that at the HLA-B locus.

The experience in London is different. Workers there found a positive and very clear correlation between compatibility for the HLA loci A and B with survival of the transplant, and it is also reported by a French group. This difference between the North American and European series is perhaps due to differences in linkage disequilibrium between some of the serological loci and those established by lymphocyte typing. There is much less experience available on HLA-D typing in cadaver transplantation. As already mentioned, these antigens are detected indirectly in mixed-lymphocyte culture (MLC), the London group has also observed a positive correlation between the degree of response in mixed-lymphocyte culture and transplant survival, but the analysis of these results would not exclude the possible influence of the HLA-A and B loci compatibility between donor and recipient.

A more important factor appears to be the compatibility between the DR antigens, according to recent reports of many cases typed for these antigens.

In conclusion, the ideal situation in kidney transplant is compatibility for the entire HLA system, but this is possible in very few cases. Moreover, if compatibility for HLA-A and B is possible, one should always consider that incompatibility for the other systems, particularly HLA-DR, is one of the possible causes of rejection, as well as the other systems recently reported. There are, however, other important factors in donor selection.

Blood groups

Blood groups of the ABO system are important in renal transplantation. Incompatibility between donor and recipient may produce an acute rejection. If it is possible, there should be exact compatibility in the ABO and rhesus systems, but there are two exceptions; O can be transplanted into A, B and AB; and Rh⁻ can be transplanted into Rh⁺.

Sex of donor and receptor

There is some information suggesting that the kidneys of male donors survive better if transplanted into multiparous women than those between women or from woman to man.

Transfusion and cross-matching

Transfusions in renal transplantation have been a problem debated for many years. On the one hand, the general consensus indicates that, by mechanisms as yet unknown, transplant survival is better in individuals who have received previous transfusions than in those who have not. In fact, most centres in the UK are now routinely performing pre-transplant transfusion. On the other hand, transfusion stimulates in the donor the formation of antibodies against antigens of the HLA system present in the lymphocytes transfused, and the selection of the donor is therefore more complicated. For this reason, the patients on chronic dialysis are studied at regular intervals for cytotoxic antibodies against a panel of lymphocytes which contain all the available HLA antigens. If it is found that the serum of the patient has antibodies against one of these antigens, a donor without that HLA type should be looked for.

In practice, individuals are frequently found who develop antibodies against many of the HLA types, and it is therefore very difficult to find a donor for these cases.

13.2. *Immunological aspects of rejection*

The immunological problems of rejection are normally divided into two phases: afferent and efferent. In the afferent phase the host recognizes the histocompatibility antigens of the transplant as foreign, and in the efferent phase generates immunological mechanisms to attack the transplant. Let us examine these two phases in more detail (See Figure 13.1).

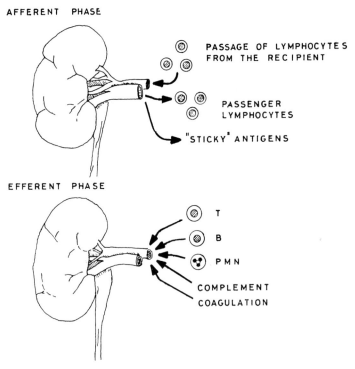

Figure 13.1. Immune mechanisms involved in the afferent and efferent phases of rejection.

Afferent phase

At least in skin grafts, lymphatic drainage is indispensable for the establishment of the afferent phase (which is also called the recognition phase). However, when vascularized organs such as the kidney are transplanted, it is not necessary for there to be lymphatic drainage and lymphatic channels of these organs to be intact for the recipient to recognize it as foreign. It is therefore clear that the afferent phase may be brought about in two ways: through the lymphatic vessels as in skin grafts, or via the blood as in the transplantation of vascularized organs.

The place in which sensitization of the recipient occurs has been long debated, and two possibilities arise: either it is in the transplant (peripheral tissue) or in the lymphatic nodes and spleen of the recipient (central). Everything seems to indicate that the lymphocytes of the recipient are sensitized while they are circulating in the transplant tissue, so that peripheral sensitization is the more probable mechanism involved in this process of recognition. This does not eliminate the other two possibilities: that there are passenger leucocytes or leucocytes from the transplanted tissue that pass from the donor to the host circulation, and that there exist 'sticky' histocompatibility antigens coming from the transplant and taken up by the recipient's cells.

Efferent phase

In this phase are generated immune mechanisms both of cellular and humoral type. In non-sensitized individuals, the cell-mediated mechanisms are the most important in rejection of the transplant. It has been suggested that at some time or another almost all the lymphoid cells are involved in cell-mediated mechanisms of rejection, including T and B lymphocytes, monocytes, 'null' lymphocytes, etc. Some of these cells have cytotoxic activities when joined by their Fc receptors to the target cells, covered with specific antibodies, by a mechanism which is known as antibody-dependent cell cytotoxicity (ADCC). The ADCC is the best known example of collaboration between antibodies and effector cells, involving macrophages, T and natural killer (NK) cells.

The most important of the cell-mediated mechanisms is, however, the direct cytotoxicity mediated by T lymphocytes of a special subpopulation, that in the mouse has been identified as $Ly1^-$, $Ly23^+$. This subpopulation makes up only 5–10% of the total of T cells. The suppressor cells, also in this group of lymphocytes, are distinguished by the presence on their surface of Ia antigens.

In the generation of these effector cells other cell groups take part. Suppressor lymphocytes may, for instance, modulate the generation of effector cells, possibly suppressing the proliferative response of T cells of type $Ly1^+$, $Ly23^-$. It is also suspected that the macrophage is of importance in the generation of effector cells.

The process of destruction of the target cells, mediated by the effector cells, may be divided into three stages: recognition, action and disintegration.

Recognition stage

It is presumed that in this stage the relation between the effector cell and the target cell is made through membrane receptors of both cells. It is also maintained that the receptors of the effector cells are directed to alloantigens of the serologically defined groups. The nature of the antigen towards which the efforts of the effector cells are directed is still not defined, so they are simply called lymphocytically defined cytolytic H antigens (LDCH).

Action stage

During this phase the effector cell acts upon the target cell to destroy it. The actual way in which the effector cell damages the target cell is unknown. Using dextran, which prevents cell interaction, it has been found that with only six minutes of interaction damage is already produced in the target cell, although the total cytolysis takes some hours. This indicates that there are mechanisms both dependent and independent of the effector T cell. On the other hand, everything seems to indicate that the receptor of the effector cell has a double function in this phase; besides being a way of recognizing the target cell, it also participates actively in the attack process, by mechanisms still difficult to define.

There are three possible ways in which the effector cell destroys the target cell:

1. The effector cells produce enzymes which destroy the membrane of the target cell.

2. The effector cells insert a protein into the membrane of the target cell, a protein which allows entry and exit of ions.

3. The effector cells secrete soluble cytotoxins.

It is not clear which of these is the more important in the process of destruction of the target cell.

Disintegration stage

Disintegration of the target cell may take several hours after its contact with the effector T cell. It has been seen that the process of disintegration of the target cell depends upon temperature, suggesting that there is an active metabolic process which needs the production of energy. However, the observations of other investigators using dextran have shown that the T cell punctures a hole approximately 9 nm in diameter in the membrane of the target cell. This perforation of the membrane would be followed by a colloidosmotic lysis.

13.3. Rejection mechanisms mediated by antibodies

Various forms of rejection are mediated by mechanisms of the humoral type, among them the hyper-acute rejection which is induced by antibodies against the antigenic determinants of the transplanted tissue. These antibodies, when joined to the antigenic determinants, activate the complement system, which generates on one hand chemotactic factors which attract the polymorphonuclear neutrophils, but on the other hand is capable of activating the coagulation system leading to the occlusion of vascularity observed in these cases.

Obviously complement will also exercise its principle function of lysis at the level perhaps of the vascular endothelium of the transplant, leading to the exposure of the subendothelium inducing even more strongly the activation of the coagulation factors.

In summary, the immune mechanisms, both cellular and humoral, are of the utmost importance in the process of tissue rejection and although the former have a clear action, the humoral system mediated by antibodies plays a predominant role at least in some cases of rejection.

13.4. Histopathology of renal rejection

Acute rejection

Acute rejection occurs during the first few days after the transplant. On about the second day a proliferation of mononuclear cells is observed in the peritubular capillaries. In the following 48–72 hours these cells pass through the capillary wall and proliferate in the renal interstitium. The capillary walls are then broken and

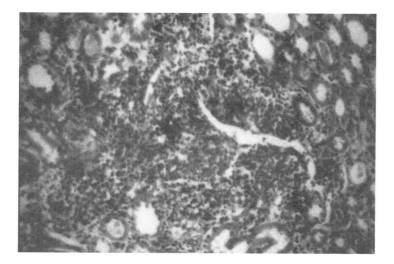

Figure 13.2. Kidney section in a case of acute rejection showing marked lymphocytic infiltration in the interstitium (courtesy of the Transplantation Group, Universidad de Antioquia, Colombia).

there is therefore ischaemia and damage of the nephron. This acute process diminishes in intensity and in a few cases may reverse with the use of immuno-suppressors, but the parenchymatous damage is irreversible and fibrous tissue replaces in time the parenchymal lesion. Also during this acute phase a fibrinoid necrosis has been observed in the arteriolae and reduplication and fibrosis of the endothelium of the larger arteries, possibly mediated by humoral antibodies (Figure 13.2).

Chronic rejection

Chronic rejection is characterized by enlargement of the intima of the arteries and arterioles with breakage of the lamina elastica interna. This is the result of the for-mation of platelet aggregates and fibrin which are deposited in the walls of the vessel and which, with the passage of time, are covered by the epithelium. In the glomerulus, the glomerular membrane is diffusely enlarged, with increase in the number of mesangeal cells and deposits of IgM, IgG, C1 and C3 similar to those observed in glomerulonephritis (Figure 13.3).

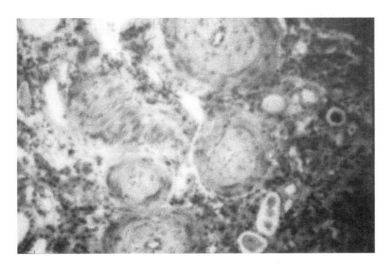

Figure 13.3. Kidney section in a case of chronic rejection showing fibrointimal prolifera-tion in small vessels and interstitial infiltration by mononuclear cells (courtesy of the Transplantation Group, Universidad de Antioquia, Colombia).

Clinical diagnosis of renal rejection

Various clinical manifestations are seen during rejection of a renal transplant, but mostly biopsy is necessary to establish the diagnosis. In histopathological examina-tion, peritubular mononuclear infiltration is considered as a specific manifestation of rejection. The measurement of plasma creatinine is also of help since any sign of acute rejection is usually accompanied by loss of renal functions. A transplant which is functioning efficiently should maintain levels of serum creatinine below 2 mg / 100 ml. Other signs of acute rejection are hyperthermia and pain in the area of the transplant, retention of liquids, diminution of urinary flow, diminution of excretion of sodium, and proteinuria. Also lymphocytosis and thrombocytopenia are frequent. An increase in the excretion of degradation products of fibrin may help in the diagnosis in the initial period of acute rejection. Also useful are signs of attenuation of the image of the small vessels in arteriography and the absence of the excretory phase on scan.

The diagnosis of chronic rejection is not so clear. Renal hypertrophy may mask the results of glomerular damage and therefore the rise in level of creatinine may be delayed. Normally there are no inflammatory signs in this type of rejection. Eventually ischaemia leads to hypertension and proteinuria.

Common causes of transplantation failure

Besides acute and chronic rejection, there are other causes of failure of renal transplant. Venous thrombosis, arterial obstruction and arterial stenosis may be observed accompanied by hypertension and haematuria. The diagnosis is made by arteriography or renal scan. In these patients all the secondary effects of the administration of immunosuppressors may be expected; of these, sepsis is the most severe and the main cause of death, particularly by infections of the respiratory tract, the genito-urinary tract and the site of surgery. The organisms most frequently found are *Escherichia coli*, *Pseudomonas aeruginosa*, *Klebsiella* and *Staphylococcus*, and the intensive treatment of these infections with antibiotics may be followed by bizarre manifestations of viral infection (cytomegalovirus, *Herpes pneumonitis*). Possibly the most adequate treatment of sepsis in the patient following renal transplantation is the suspension of immunosuppression, allowing his own immune system to recover, although this puts at risk the success of the transplant.

Immunosuppression

Four principal agents are used as immunosuppressors in the post-operative management of a renal transplant: corticosteroids, cyclosporin, azathioprine and antilymphocytic serum or globulin. In large doses the corticoids may produce a pronounced diminution in the number of circulating lymphocytes and in the levels of immunoglobulin G. In acute rejection, their use frequently reverses the process, but necessitates very high doses (up to 1 g/kg of methylprednisolone per day). It is necessary therefore to restrict the period of administration to the minimum; usually four to five days are sufficient. If there are no manifestations of rejection, it is recommended to start with 1–2 mg/kg/day and to reduce the doses in a few weeks to less toxic levels. Azathioprine is one of the imidazole derivatives of 6-mercaptopurine much used in renal transplantations. It has the disadvantage of producing sudden bone-marrow depression. Adequate doses (usually around 1.5–3.0 mg/kg/day) should be prescribed in accordance with renal function, since this is important for its detoxification.

Antilymphocytic globulin is also used in various centres in association with steroids. Possibly renal function is better in patients who receive this type of treatment but this is still debatable. Cyclosporin A, a peptide fungal metabolite, is the most promising new immunosuppressor. Although it is nephrotoxic, its use seems to improve graft survival.

13.5. Bone-marrow transplants

Bone marrow contains cells which have the capacity to differentiate into haematopoetic, phagocytic, megakaryocytic and lymphoid, so therefore the transplant of bone marrow should provide precursors of all these systems. Table 13.1 lists the disorders in which this type of transplant has been most successful.

Table 13.1. Diseases in which a bone-marrow transplantation should be considered.

Severe combined immunodeficiency
Aplastic anaemia
Wiskott–Aldrich syndrome
Myeloid and lymphoid acute leukaemias
Chronic granulomatosis
C1q deficiency
Congenital neutropenia

General aspects

Various methods of pre-transplant treatment are used in order to reduce the risk of rejection. Cyclophosphamide at doses of 45 mg/kg daily intravenously during the four days before the transplant is perhaps the method used most. Whole-body radiation has also been suggested with 950–1000 rads, and other groups have made use of various combinations of anti-lymphocytic globulin and methotrexate.

Graft-versus-host disease

This reaction is the result of the immunological process mounted by the transplanted lymphoid tissue against the tissue of the recipient. Clinically it is characterized by hepatomegaly, splenomegaly, weight loss, nausea, vomiting, diarrhoea, anaemia and exfoliative dermatitis. The degree of diarrhoea and dermatitis is used to assess the severity of the reaction. The major complication of this reaction is infection certainly due to the profound immunological depression which follows it.

Graft-versus-host reaction is observed in every transplant of bone marrow or fetal liver, but it is of moderate extent between HLA-identical sibs and increases in severity with the incompatibility between donor and recipient.

Procedure

Transplantation of bone marrow is in itself a simple procedure. Under general anaesthesia 300–500 ml of bone marrow are aspirated from the iliac crest of the donor and placed in a heparinized sterile flask. After filtration of this material in order to remove bone spicules that may remain after the surgery, it is applied intravenously into the recipient at a very slow rate.

Donor selection

Compatibility for the HLA system is always more important in this type of transplant than in renal. Of all the loci of the system, the most decisive appears to be the HLA-D region although the others must obviously contribute to the success or rejection.

Taking into account the compatibility in the HLA system and the familial relationship between donor and recipient, all the cases of bone-marrow transplantation so far carried out may be classified into four groups.

1. A transplant coming from an HLA genotypically identical sib.
2. A transplant from another relative compatible for the HLA system.
3. A transplant coming from an individual compatible for the HLA system but not related to the recipient.
4. A transplant coming from unrelated individuals incompatible for the HLA system with the recipient.

Let us look at each of these groups separately.

Transplantation from a genotypically identical sib

Many patients with severe combined immunodeficiency have received a transplant from a sib identical in the HLA system. The results are excellent and show a total re-establishment of the functions of T and B cells, a low intensity of graft-versus-host reaction, and survival of the patients for up to 10 years. In these patients a chimeric phenomenon is probably present, as in a case described in 1975 of a girl with a severe combined immunodeficiency and a deficiency of the enzyme adenosine deaminase (ADA). The transplant was donated by her sister who had normal concentrations of ADA. Later studies showed that the erythrocytes of the patient were still deficient in the enzyme while all the other lymphoid cells produced it normally.

There is less experience available from treatment of the Wiskott–Aldrich syndrome. It seems that at the beginning the haematopoietic anomalies did not improve with the transplant, but in more recent cases complete haematological and immunological reconstitution has been obtained by the use of anti-thymocytic globulin and whole-body radiation before the transplant.

Transplantation from an HLA-compatible relative

Due to the small size of European and American families, it is not always possible to find a sib compatible with the patient. In these cases other relatives are studied and the graft is taken from the one with the greatest genetic similarity to the recipient. This means that frequently not all of the antigens of the HLA-A and B systems are the same in the donor and recipient, but compatibility at the HLA-D and DR loci are of the utmost importance in determining the donor.

Table 13.2 shows the results of some of the cases in which genetically identical sibs have not been used, but in which the donor was chosen from among the near relatives of the patient. The results of this type of transplant are not so acceptable, but a definite rejection has not been observed and a total or partial reconstitution has been obtained.

Table 13.2.

Donor	Incompat. HLA	Reconst. cell. A	Reconst. cell. B	Reference
Father	None	+	+	Polmar & Sorensen (1976)
Father	None	±	−	Geha *et al.* (1976)
Father	None	+	+	Anderson (1975)
Uncle	None	+	No	Vossen *et al.* (1973)
Uncle	B	+	−	Copenhagen (1973)
Mother	A	+	±	Niethammer *et al.* (1976)
Father	A	+	+	Copenhagen (1976)

Transplantation from an unrelated compatible donor

Several cases of this type are already known. One of them received bone marrow from a donor who differed only in a single HLA antigen but who was compatible in mixed-lymphocyte culture. Unfortunately the patient died a month after the transplant from an interstitial pneumonia and it was not possible to assess in such a short time the immunological reaction. Another patient required seven grafts from a donor compatible for HLA-B and D, but not identical for HLA-A before definite immunological function was established. This type of transplant may potentially be very useful, but it is necessary to increase the number of possible donors of known HLA type and include all this information in a local computerized system which permits access to the correct donor at the critical time.

Transplantation from an incompatible donor

This group includes the patients who have received grafts of bone marrow from donors who are not compatible or those who have received transplants of other tissues, and in whom various methods have been used to reduce the intensity of the graft-versus-host reaction. The object of these methods is to eliminate from the transplanted tissue the lymphoid cells that will create the rejection reaction. This has been obtained by a purely physical separation, either using gradients of serum bovine albumin or by sedimentation rate, but other methods have also been tried, such as treatment of the tissue with anti-lymphocytic serum, 5-bromodeoxyuridine and tritiated thymidine, without good results. In the same way foetal tissues have been used for transplant of liver and thymus in the treatment of severe combined immunodeficiency when an adequate donor has not been found to provide a bone-marrow graft.

The prognosis of this type of treatment has improved since the use of fresh cells, foetal donors of less than 13 weeks' gestation, and a second transplant where there is no immunological reconstitution three months after the first. It seems that other factors like the number of cells and the route of administration, which were formerly considered important, are not so crucial. In the variants of severe combined immunodeficiency with thymic aplasia the combined use of foetal thymus and liver is indicated.

13.6. Transplants of other organs

Liver transplants

Liver transplant is considered in any patient with terminal liver disease, without infection or generalized malignant disease and less than 50 years of age.

The liver appears to be more resistant to rejection than kidney. The presence of cytotoxic antibodies in the recipient and incompatibility of the ABO blood groups which are important in renal transplantation have not been shown to increase the rejection reaction of the liver. There is insufficient information to assess the importance of the HLA system, since the majority of the transplants so far carried out have not received tissue compatible for their system. Besides the surgical problems, the main causes of failure of liver transplants are rejection and infection. Rejection is characterized by icterus from the first post-transplant week with increased levels of alkaline phosphatase, transaminase and bilirubin. There has been described a slow form which may take two to four weeks and an anicteroid form. The post-operative immunosuppression is very similar to that used in renal transplants, but taking into account the fact that azathioprine is hepatotoxic, and it must therefore be carefully controlled. Bacterial and fungal infections have been reported in these patients.

The diagnosis of rejection is not easy since the tests of hepatic function are not specific. Nowadays hepatic biopsy is used, as well as colangiography and the leucocyte migration test.

Heart transplants

Until 1978, 406 heart transplants had been carried out throughout the world on 395 patients, of which almost 25% were carried out in 1968 when this surgical technique was first developed.

Although the prognosis in this type of transplant has not greatly improved (50% survive one year post-transplant), it is possible that the new tendencies in the groups active in this field may be followed by more positive results in the future. For instance, the contra-indications were not closely defined. In the light of experience, four absolute contra-indications have been defined: severe pulmonary hypertension, systemic infections, insulin-dependent diabetes, and cytotoxic antibodies in the recipient.

The acute rejection, which is still the major problem, is now being diagnosed early by transvenous endomyocardial biopsy. The typical histopathological findings are polymorphonuclear infiltration, interstitial oedema and cytolysis of the myocardial fibres. A late complication is the development of coronary arteriosclerosis in the transplant, which presents between three months and six years post-operatively and the control of this is receiving much attention.

Skin transplant

Although this was the first organ to be transplanted (at the beginning of the nineteenth century there were already autotransplants), the survival of skin allotransplants is even more difficult to obtain than that of the kidney, and the compatibility of the HLA system plays a role of the utmost importance.

Skin transplants may be utilized sometimes in the treatment of severe burns. As early as 1974 this type of transplant was carried out using skin from fathers to treat their children with burns, combining it with autotransplants as well. With the use of antithymocytic globulin these allotransplants survive up to six weeks diminishing the loss of liquid and proteins, reducing the risk of infection and giving sufficient time for the complete replacement with autotransplants.

Pancreas transplants

Two classes of pancreatic transplant have been tried: (a) the complete or the majority of the organ, and (b) the endocrine component. Various surgical forms have been tried for transplanting part of the complete organ:

1. Pancreatic duodenal transplant.
2. Transplant of the body and tail of the pancreas with anastamosis of the duct to the ureter of the recipient or a non-functional intestinal loop.

3. A complete transplant with ligature of the duct.
4. Complete transplant and obstruction of the duct with neoprene rubber.

With these techniques some satisfactory results have been obtained, but besides the surgical complications there are frequent secondary problems due to the accumulation of enzymes of the exocrine drainage of the organ. The alternative is to transplant the endocrine component which may be separated by physical measures, suspended in solution and injected via the portal vein to become disseminated in the liver.

The techniques of separating the islet cells are not complicated, but the problem is that an adult pancreas will produce less than 10% of the total mass of islets and this is not sufficient to produce a significant change in the diabetes in the recipients. With the object of increasing the quantity of cells, foetal pancreas has been tried, which, if taken sufficiently early in gestation before the exocrine component has developed, can be transplanted without the necessity of separating the islet cells.

Some 160 transplants of islet cells have been performed, and the results of most of them are known. None has shown any significant improvement.

Other groups have tried intra-splenic implantation instead of hepatic, the result being that the spleen tolerates without complications large quantities of pancreatic enzymes, which suggests that this may be a better site for the transplantation of cellular suspensions. Recently we have tried gut intra-parietal implantation in dogs without complications.

Rejection

As in every organ, rejection is a serious problem in pancreatic transplantation. The islet cells transplanted into histo-incompatible individuals are inactivated within two to three days. To avoid rejection, some investigators have experimented with β-cell cultures in membranes permeable to insulin which are implanted as small tubes in blood vessels. Although theoretically possible, there would be secondary problems like thrombosis, replacement or excessive propagation of β cells.

In summary, pancreatic transplantation is still highly experimental and its place in the treatment of diabetes is far from clear.

Bibliography

Anderson, I. M., Bone marrow transplants. *Proc. R. Soc. Med.*, **68**: 577 (1975).
Biggar, W. D. and Park, R. A., Compatible bone marrow transplantation and immunologic reconstitution of combined immunodeficiency disease. *Birth Defects*, **11**: 385 (1975).
Clarkson, B. D., Current concepts in leukemia and results of recent treatment programs. *Transplant. Proc.*, **10**: 157 (1978).

Copenhagen Study Group of Immunodeficiencies, Bone marrow transplantation from an HLA-non-identical but mixed-lymphocyte-culture identical donor. *Lancet*, ii: 791 (1973).

Diethelm, A. G., Dimick, A. R., Shaw, J. F., Baker, H. J. and Phillips, S. J., Treatment of a severely burned child with transplantation modified by immunosuppressive therapy. *Ann. Surg.*, **180**: 814 (1974).

Geha, R. S., Malakian, A., LeFranc, G., Chayban, D. and Serre, J. L., Immunologic reconstitution in severe combined immunodeficiency following transplantation with parental bone marrow. *Pediatrics*, **58**: 451 (1976).

Griepp, R. B., A decade of human heart transplantation. *Transplant. Proc.*, 111: 285 (1979).

Hamburger, J., Clinical transplantation. *Transplant. Proc.*, 11: 1 (1979).

Horowitz, S. D., Bach, F. H. and Groshong, T., Treatment of severe combined immunodeficiency with bone marrow from unrelated, mixed leukocyte-culture-non-reactive donor. *Lancet*, i: 431 (1975).

Morris, P. J., Matching for HLA in transplantation. *Br. Med. Bull.*, **34**: 259 (1978).

Najarian, J. S. and Ascher, N. L., Causes and management of rejection. *Transplant. Proc.*, **11**: 11 (1979).

Niethammer, D., Goldman, S. F. and Haas, R. J., Bone marrow transplantation for severe combined immunodeficiency with the HLA-A incompatible but MLC-identical mother as donor. *Transplant. Proc.*, **8**: 623 (1976).

Opelz, G., Gale, R. P., Feig, S. A'., Walker, J., Terasaki, P. I. and Saxon, A. and the UCLA Bone Marrow Transplant Team, Significance of HLA and non-HLA antigens in bone marrow transplantation. *Transplant. Proc.*, **10**: 43 (1978).

O'Reilly, R. J., Pahwa, R. and Pahwa, S., Fetal tissue transplantation in severe combined immunodeficiency. In *International Cooperative Group for Bone Marrow Transplantation in Man*. Third Workshop, Tarrytown, N. Y. (1976).

Pahwa, R., Pahwa, S., O'Reilly, R. and Good, R., Treatment of immunodeficiency diseases — Progress toward replacement therapy emphasizing cellular and macromolecular engineering. *Springer Seminars in Immunopathology*, 1: 355 (1978).

Pober, J. S., Collins, T., Gimbrone, J. A., Cotron, R. S., Gitlin, J. D., Fiers, W., Clayberger, C., Krensky, A. M., Burakoff, S. J. and Reiss, C. S., Lymphocytes recognise human vascular endothelial and dermal fibroblast Ia antigens induced by recombinant immune interferon. *Nature*, **305**: 726 (1983).

Polmar, S. and Sorensen, R. U., Parent–child bone marrow transplant in severe immunodeficiency. In *International Cooperative Group for Bone Marrow Transplantation in Man*. Third Workshop, Tarrytown, N.Y. (1976).

Solheim, B. G., The role of pretransplant blood transfusion. *Transplant. Proc.*, **11**: 138 (1979).

Starzl, T. E., Koep, J., Halgrimson, C. G., Hood, J., Schroter, G. P. J., Porter, K. A. and Weil III, R., Liver transplantation. *Transplant. Proc.*, 11: 240 (1979).

Taylor, R. M. R., Ting, A. and Briggs, J. D., Renal transplantation in the United Kingdom and Ireland — the centre effect. *Lancet*, i: 789 (1985).

Vossen, J. M., de Koning, J. and van Bekkum, D. W., Successful treatment of an infant with severe combined immunodeficiency by transplantation of bone marrow cells from an uncle. *Clin. Exp. Immunol.*, **13**: 20 (1973).

Williams, G. M., Progress in clinical renal transplantation. *Transplant. Proc.*, 11: 4 (1979).

Zeitz, H. J., Gewurz, A., Jonasson, O., Gris, W. P. and Gewurz, H., Renal transplantation in a patient with hereditary deficiency of the second component of complement. *Clin. Exp. Immunol.*, **46**: 420 (1981).

Chapter 14. Immunogenetics and the human gene map

Preceding chapters have given an overall view of the genetic aspects of the immune system and its clinical applications. The purpose of the present chapter is to summarize present-day knowledge on the location of genes involved in the immune response, and then describe a miscellanea of defects and concepts associated with the chromosome complement, or with a possible Mendelian pattern of inheritance.

14.1. The assignment of genes to specific chromosomes

There are several ways by which genes are usually allocated to particular chromosomes. The pattern of inheritance of alternative forms of a single characteristic, or of a disorder, almost always permits the identification of those genes that are situated on chromosome X. This was the first step in the assignment of genes to human chromosomes, and today therefore the map of the X chromosome is very well known. If the gene in question is not on the X chromosome it may be situated on any one of the 22 pairs of autosomes and it is not always easy to define which. In these cases it is possible to use markers — genes of a known location on a specific chromosome. By examining the pattern of transmission of the gene in question and the marker gene, whether or not they are close on the same chromosome can be established. This not only allows the chromosome to be identified, but it also allows the distance between the two genes on the same chromosome to be measured, according to the frequency with which they recombine. This method seems simple, but it requires numerous families in which the mating types in respect of the two genes are informative, and these are not always easy to find.

Undoubtedly the human gene map has developed very much since the introduction of sophisticated laboratory techniques which allow cell fusion between different species. These techniques are generally known as cell hybridization techniques, for they simply allow the incorporation of one or more human chromosomes in say the cell of a mouse, followed by study of the biochemical products of this new hybrid cell. Since the chromosomes of mouse and man are easily distinguishable under the microscope, and their products can be identified, the concurrence of a given chromosome and a given product indicates that the gene coding for the product is on that particular chromosome. Many of the gene locations which we now have, have been established by this method.

A rapidly developing method is that of DNA probes, whereby particular DNA sequences are identified and gene location in relation to these follows in the same way as with marker genes.

There are other methods, such as the Lepore method and genetic dosage, which are worth mentioning but do not need to be reviewed here.

Assignment of genes associated with the immune system

Figure 14.1 shows diagrammatically the distribution of the genes associated with the immune system; a list of these is given in Table 14.1. Undoubtedly the best known are those controlling the great variety of blood groups. The genes of the ABO system are located on chromosome 9 on its long arm, linked to the adenylate kinase locus; the Rh blood-group genes are on chromosome 1 on the short arm and linked to one of the loci of elliptocytosis and to 6PGD; the genes for Dombrock and Duffy blood groups are also on chromosome 1, the genes for blood group P on chromosome 6 on its long arm, Colton and Kidd on chromosome 7, and Xg on chromosome X.

On chromosome 1 and chromosome 17 three sites have been identified which are particularly susceptible to the action of the adenovirus 12. These are known as modification sites of adenovirus 12.

It seems that the production of interferon requires several loci, one of them on chromosome 2 and the other on chromosome 5 or perhaps chromosome 9. One of these may be the structural gene while the other may encode for a specific receptor, necessary for the activation of the structural gene. There are, however, two other possibilities: both genes may code for subunits of the interferon molecule, or one may code for a precursor form of interferon and the other may be involved in its activation. More recent data involve chromosomes 12 and 13 in the synthesis of some form of interferon. Besides these loci another may also exist, possibly on chromosome 16, producing a depressor of the anti-viral state induced by interferon, and there is possibly also another on chromosome 21 producing an antiviral protein mediating the inhibition of viral replication induced by interferon.

Sensitivity to various viruses and toxins has been assigned to genes within the human genome. Among these susceptibility to herpes has been assigned to a gene on chromosome 3. Cell hybrids between human and mouse have led to the suggestion that susceptibility to polio virus depends on a gene on chromosome 19, possibly encoding for a receptor for the polio virus. Another possibly distinct gene but on the same chromosome may determine cell sensitivity to echo virus 11.

On chromosome 5 there is a gene which probably produces a receptor for

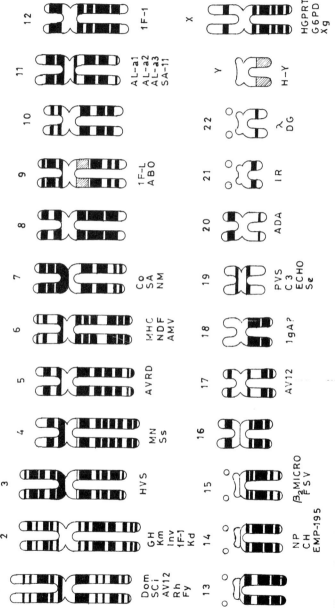

Figure 14.1. Chromosome assignment of genes related to the immune system (see list in Table 14.1).

Table 14.1. Location of genes associated with the immune system.

Chromosome 1
Rhesus blood group (*Rh*)
Scianna blood group (*Sci*)
Dombrock blood group (*Dom*)
Duffy blood group (*Fy*)
Adenovirus-12 modification site (*AV-12*)

Chromosome 2
Interferon 1 (*IF-1*)
Immunoglobulin heavy-chain attachment site (*CH*)
Immunoglobulin kappa light-chain gene family (*Km, Inv*)
Kidd blood group (*Kd*)

Chromosome 3
Herpes virus sensitivity (*HVS*)

Chromosome 4
MN blood group (*MN*)
Ss blood group (*Ss*)

Chromosome 5
Antiviral state repressor regulator (*AVRD*)

Chromosome 6
Major histocompatibility complex (*MHC*)
Neutrophil differentiation factor (*NDF*)
Oncogene : avian myeloblastosis virus (*AMV*)

Chromosome 7
Colton blood group (*CO*)
Neutrophil migration (*NM*)
Surface antigen 6 (*SA*)

Chromosome 9
Leucocyte interferon gene family (*IF-L*)
ABO blood group (*ABO*)

Chromosome 11
Surface antigens A1–14

Chromosome 12
Interferon, immune type (*IF-I*)

Chromosome 14
External membrane protein 195 (*EMP-195*)
Immunoglobulin heavy-chain gene family (*CH*)
Nucleoside phosphorylase (*NP*)

Chromosome 15
Mz — microglobulin
Oncogene : feline sarcoma virus (*FSV*)

Chromosome 17
Adenovirus-12 modification site (*AV-12*)

Chromosome 19
Polio virus sensitivity (*PVS*)
Echo-11 sensitivity (*ECHO*)
Complement component 3 (*C3*)
Secretor (*Se*)

Chromosome 20
Adenosine deaminase (*ADA*)

Chromosome 21
Interferon receptor (*IR*)

Table 14.1 continued

Chromosome 22
Di George Syndrome (*DG*)
Immunoglobulin lambda light-chain gene family (λ)
Chromosome X
Xg blood group
G6PD
HGPRT
Chromosome Y
H-Y antigen

---

diphtheria toxin. This toxin is composed of a polypeptide chain with two fragments, one the effector and the other the haptomere responsible for its union with the cell surface.

At least four cell-surface antigens have been associated with the same number of chromosomes, all of them detected by somatic cell studies. Their importance is still unknown.

On chromosome 11 there has been identified a locus which controls the expression of a surface antigen, named 'killer' or 'lethal' antigen by some. It seems that this lethal antigen is a genetic complex consisting of at least three loci, which may correspond to those described as A1, A2 and A3 from the FA1 system. A similarity has been suggested between A1 and glycophorin which is the main surface glycoprotein of the human red cells, in the amino terminal portion of which are located the oligosaccharides which determine the blood group antigens.

The location of the loci which control structural variations of the immunoglobulin molecule are now established. The human immunoglobulin genes are located on chromosomes 22 (λ chains), 2 ($\varkappa$ chains) and 14 (H chain). The Km system has also been located together with the Kidd and Colton groups.

There has been observed a congenital neutropenia associated with HLA B12 possibly in linkage disequilibrium, and this has led to the suggestion that there is a gene controlling the differentiation of the neutrophil, linked to the MHS on chromosome 6. On the other hand a case of monosomy 7 with chemotactic defects has also been observed, suggesting that there may be a gene controlling the normal chemotactic response of the neutrophils on this chromosome.

Among the enzymes important in the immune system, the gene of nucleoside phosphorylase has been assigned by cell hybridization to chromosome 14. This enzyme was shown to be molecularly heterogeneous since two children were observed in a single family with activity of less than 1% of this enzyme, but both parents carried different electrophoretic mutants. The locus of adenosine deaminase has been identified on chromosome 20. This enzyme has three common phenotypes designated ADA1, ADA21 and ADA2. A locus of hypoxanthine guanine phosphoribosyl transferase has been located on the X chromosome by means of somatic cell studies; absence of this enzyme produces the Lesch-Nyhan syndrome.

14.2. Concepts and immunological defects with a genetic or chromosomal base

The chromosome complement and IgM levels

Susceptibility to bacterial infections is greater in men than in women, which suggests that this difference is of genetic origin and mediated by the number of X chromosomes. However, the study of normal populations shows a difference consistent only in the IgM levels; the women normally have higher levels of IgM than men. Our experience is very similar. Studies of adults of both sexes and of different ethnic origins show a quite consistent difference in IgM levels. However, in a recent sample of newborn infants we observed a difference in IgG levels also, for which there is no explanation.

Although the sex variation in IgM levels may in principle be attributed to genetic effects, many other factors are also probably involved. These have been examined in the mouse with different chromosome complements, among which are occasional individuals 39X0 (a mouse Turner), and individuals karyotypically of both sexes but with the gene *Sxr* which has been mentioned already. These findings confirm the existence of higher levels of IgM in females, and a similar difference has been observed in humans. On the other hand, the 39X0 mice had no lower levels than the normal 40XX, and the levels in the animals 40XY; 40XX, Sxr + ; and 40XY, Sxr + do not show significant differences, suggesting that the difference in IgM levels in the two sexes is perhaps more of hormonal rather than purely genetic origin.

The chromosome complement and the levels of alphafoetoprotein

It was thought for a time that there was a sex difference in the AFP levels in cord blood. Since it was suggested that AFP may have some immuno-suppressor effect, a sex difference in levels at birth would possibly contribute to the greater susceptibility of males to infections of bacterial type. However, this suppressor effect could not be shown *in vivo*, and neither could any sex difference in AFP levels in cord blood be established between the two sexes.

Inheritance of anti-thyroid antibodies

In the past 10 years it has become evident that there is a familial component in the presence of antibodies against the components of the thyroid gland. However, it is much more difficult to define the mechanisms of inheritance. In several studies relatives of patients with thyroid disease of auto-immune type have been found with antibodies but without the disease. It has even been suggested that a single gene could control this predisposition. The last study of this topic has done much to clarify the situation. In a family study covering 322 individuals a higher incidence of relatives with antibodies was indeed observed but without a clear pattern of inheritance, and the authors therefore suggested that the capacity to form anti-thyroid antibodies has a multifactorial mode of inheritance with a moderate heritability (up to 53%). For several of the auto-immune diseases of the thyroid there is therefore a susceptibility to the formation of antibodies, and this could eventually prove applicable to other types of auto-immune pathology.

Down's syndrome

Patients with Down's syndrome have a pronounced tendency to develop recurrent infections and disorders of a malignant type. These facts have led various investigators to study the immune system in patients with this trisomy, and they report cellular and humoral anomalies. Some of these patients also have hyperuricaemia, which suggests that they may also have an anomaly of purine metabolism.

In general patients with Down's syndrome also have higher levels of IgG than the controls of the same sex and age. Besides this, they do not have an adequate reaction to many of the antigens employed in cutaneous hypersensitivity reactions; many of them do not react with *Candida albicans*, PPD and DNCB, which suggests that there is a defect in the afferent arm of the immune response.

Some of the defects, at the level of purine metabolism, manifest themselves as immunodeficiency (amongst these can be included the Lesch-Nyhan syndrome which is accompanied by a minor defect of humoral immunity). It has however been observed that the hyperuricaemia and immune defects in Down's syndrome are independent of each other. Other studies of immune function in Down's syndrome have confirmed these findings, and also suggest that these patients have low levels of IgM and a pronounced diminution of the chemotactic response of neutrophils. However, the severity of the immune defect seems not to be related to any history of infections in these patients, so its importance in the natural history of the disease remains controversial.

Turner's syndrome

Three cases have been observed of a variant of Turner's syndrome where there is an isochromosome (karyotype 46X, i (Xq)) in which the long arm is duplicated. These three patients all showed selective deficiency of IgA. There is so far no explanation of these findings.

Acquired granulomatous disease

At the Fourth International Congress of Human Genetics a case was reported of an adult patient with chronic granulomatous ulceration of the perineum, a defect in chemotaxis and intracellular killing of the polymorphonuclear neutrophils. The chromosome study showed a tetraploid cell line with a structural aberration of chromosome 16.

Myotonic dystrophy

Myotonic dystrophy is a disease which is transmitted as an autosomal dominant and which develops with dystrophic changes in muscular tissue, leading to muscular weakness, atrophy and myotonia. Other systems are also involved and one frequently sees testicular atrophy, early frontal baldness, cataracts and excessive production of insulin. Although the basic immunological defect in this disease is unknown, the levels of IgG are usually low, due to excessive catabolism of this immunoglobulin. The measurement of IgG levels is therefore important in the diagnosis of this disease, in conjunction with slit lamp examination and electromyography.

Chromosomal disorders in immunodeficiency (Swiss type)

It seems that a single case of this type of immunodeficiency has been reported together with a chromosomal study. In this patient breakage of chromosomes and chromatids was found, and also a deficiency of C1q of the complement system. Also a high incidence of chromosomal breakage occurs in other diseases in which there is a higher susceptibility to develop infections and malignancies. Such is the case in Bloom's syndrome, Fanconi's anaemia and ataxia telangiectasia. As is well known, some viruses produce chromosomal rupture both *in vivo* and *in vitro*, and this may explain these findings.

Other immunodeficiencies associated with chromosomal disorders

IgA deficiency has sometimes been associated with anomalies of chromosome 18, particularly deletions of either arm, ring forms and enlarged chromosomes. Recently four families with immunodeficiency and chromosome anomalies were investigated, and among them was an inversion of chromosome 7, translocation of chromosomes 13 and 18, large satellites on chromosome 21 and a mosaic 45XX,−18/46XX, r18. In all of these were observed severe deficiency of one or more of the immunoglobulins and minor somatic abnormalities. A case of rheumatoid arthritis has been reported in a girl with a deletion of chromosome 18 (18p^-) but with normal levels of all the immunoglobulins including IgA.

Cytogenetics in auto-immune haemolytic anaemia

A study of 19 children with auto-immune haemolytic anaemia showed in all of them at least one chromosomal abnormality. This suggests that the etiological agents associated with auto-immune haemolytic anaemia affect the chromosomal apparatus, which is an accordance with possible viral activity. However, it is possible that an abnormal chromosomal constitution may be one of the predisposing factors to auto-immune haemolytic anaemia.

Thrombocytopenia

There are two defects of platelets, besides the Wiskott-Aldrich syndrome, associated with immune dysfunction. In sex-linked essential thrombocytopenia there occur low or absent levels of isohaemaglutinins and high levels of IgA. However, another form of thrombocytopenia has been described, with high levels of IgA and renal disease (glomerulonephritis) possibly sex linked.

Other conditions

Hereditary nephropathy and deafness (Alport's syndrome) seems to be an autosomal dominant. It has been shown that the serum of these patients is capable of inactivating C3 *in vitro*, and in Japan anti-thyroid antibodies have been found in the serum of many of these patients. Therefore it has been suggested that this syndrome may be an immunological defect.

Patients with familial cold urticaria develop severe urticaria, fever and joint pain at low temperatures. The disease is inherited as an autosomal dominant. It is perhaps due to liberation by cold of histamine and chemotactic factors.

Meltzer's syndrome shows cryoglobulinaemia with systemic manifestations. A case of a woman and four of her children with a pattern of autosomal dominant inheritance has been reported.

There is a recorded case of a Negro family with a type of congenital inherited dyskeratosis which is different from normal in that it shows autosomal dominant inheritance. These individuals present with anaemia, palmar hyperkeratosis, osteoporosis, absence of dermatoglyphs and an immunological problem possibly of the afferent arm.

Hereditary neutrophilia is a benign disorder, possibly dominant, in which the neutrophilia persists throughout life, with symptoms being hepatosplenomegaly, Gaucher-type histiocytes and enlargement of the cranial dipole. A single family is known.

Various cases of familial eosinophilia have been described which are very probably inherited as an autosomal dominant.

A single familial case of disorder in the assembly of IgA is known. A woman, her mother and her son did not assemble the heavy and light chains of IgA that instead circulated freely in the serum. This is probably an autosomal dominant.

The May-Hegglin anomaly, inherited as an autosomal dominant, consists of a combination of giant platelets and leucocytes with cytoplasmic inclusion bodies known as Döhle's bodies. These bodies are actually crystalline forms of D-polymerized ribosomes, and are also seen in patients with acute myeloblastic leukaemia.

In the Pelger-Huet anomaly the nucleus of the granulocytes is less segmented and has a curious peanut shape. The anomaly is inherited as an autosomal dominant and has also been observed in a family with proximal muscular dystrophy. It is a curious fact that this anomaly is also found in the rabbit, in which the homozygous state is accompanied by a form of chondrodystrophy.

There are at least five studies of families with the triad asthma, nasal polyps and aspirin intolerance, some suggesting recessive inheritance and others dominant. It seems that the majority of cases are nevertheless sporadic without any familial antecedent. Another form of asthma appeared in one family associated with short stature and high levels of IgA.

Several cases of neuronal dysplasia with cellular immunodeficiency, which is very possibly inherited as an autosomal recessive, have been described. The neurological disorder appears to be the result of a defect in neuronal migration during embryogenesis. By contrast with ataxia telangiectasia, the levels of immunoglobulins are normal in this entity.

Immunological disorders occur in Bloom's syndrome, a rare disease inherited as an autosomal recessive which is characterized by a telangiectasic erythema in the face (usually starting early in life), hypersensitivity to sunlight and small stature. In this entity there is an increased incidence of leukaemia which seems to be related to the multiple chromosome breakages that are usually observed. The immune response of the lymphocytes in these patients is quite abnormal *in vitro*, and low circulating levels of IgA and IgM have frequently been observed.

Another defect, very possibly recessive, and observed so far in a single family, is the nephrotic syndrome, chondroitin sulphaturia and immunodeficiency. The immune defect is perhaps in the cellular arm.

Bibliography

Adinolfi, M., Haddad, S. A. and Seller, M. J., X chromosome complement and serum level of IgM in man and mouse *J. Immunogenet.*, **5**: 149 (1978).

Bernal, J. E. and Wagstaff, T. I., Cord serum AFP and the immunological status of the mother: a lack of correlation. *Biol. Neonate*, **37**: 297 (1980).

Bjorksten, B., Back, O., Hagglof, B. and Tarnvik, A., Immune function in Down's syndrome. In *Inborn Errors of Immunity and Phagocytosis*, edited by F. Guttler, J. W. T. Seakins and R. A. Harkness. MTP Press Limited, Lancaster (1979).

Boyd. E., Ferguson-Smith, M. A., Peebles-Brown, D. A., Singh, H. and Wilkinson, P. C., Acquired granulomatous disease: a hitherto undescribed condition associated with a presumptive chromosomal mutation in the bone marrow. *Excerpta Medica. International Congress Series*, No. 233: 33 (1971).

Caballero, C., Veremans, N., Lopez del Campo, J. G. and Robyn, C., Serum alpha-fetoprotein in adults, in women during pregnancy, in children at birth, and during the first week of life: a sex difference. *Am. J. Obstet. Gynecol.*, **127**: 384 (1977).

Candy, D. C. A., Hayward, A. R., Hughes, D. T., Layward, L. and Soothill, J. F., Four families with immunodeficiency and chromosome abnormalities. *Arch. Dis. Child.*, **54**: 518 (1979).

Cohn, J., Hauge, M., Andersen, V., Kenningsen, K., Nielsen, L. S., Thomsen, M. and Iversen, T., Sex-linked hereditary thrombocytopenia with immunological defects. *Hum. Hered.*, **25**: 309 (1975).

Finley, W. H., Johnson, J. C., Finley, S. C. and Dodson, W. H., Rheumatoid arthritis in a female child with a chromosome 18 deletion syndrome (46,XX, 18p). *Excerpta Medica. International Congress Series*, No. 233: 67 (1971).

Gutenberger, J., Trygstad, C. W., Steihm, E. R., Opitz, J. M., Thatcher, L. G. and Bloodworth, J. M., Familial thrombocytopenia, elevated serum IgA levels and renal disease. A report of a kindred. *Am. J. Med.*, **49**: 729(1970).

Hall, R., Dingle, P. R. and Roberts, D. F., Thyroid antibodies: study of first degree relatives. *Clin. Genet.*, **3**: 319 (1972).

Herring, W. B., Smith, L. G., Walker, R. I. and Heriom, J. C., Hereditary neutrophilia. *Am. J. Med.*, **56**: 729 (1974).

Hutteroth, T. H., Litwin, S. D. and German, J., Abnormal immune responses of Bloom's syndrome lymphocytes *in vitro*. *J. Clin. Invest.*, **56**: 1 (1975).

Jacobs, J. C., Blanc, W. A., Capoa, A., Heird, W. C., McGilvray, E., Miller, O. J., Morse, J. H., Rossen, R. D., Schullinger, J. N. and Walzer, R. A., Complement deficiency and chromosomal breaks in a case of Swiss-type agammaglobulinemia. *Lancet*, i: 499 (1968).

Lockey, R. I., Rucknagel, D. L. and Vanselow, N. A., Familial occurrence of asthma, nasal polyps and aspirin intolerance. *Ann. Intern. Med.*, **78**: 57 (1973).

McKusick, V. A. and Ruddle, F. H., The status of the gene map of the human chromosomes. *Science*, **196**: 190 (1977).

Meltzer, M. and Franklin, E. C., Cryoglobulinemia — a clinical and laboratory study. *Am. J. Med.*, **40**: 837 (1966).

Miyoshi, K., Suzuki, M., Ohno, F., Yamano, T., Yagi, F. and Khono, H., Antithyroid antibodies in Alport's syndrome. *Lancet*, ii: 480 (1975).

Moroz, C., Amir, J. and Devries, A., A hereditary immunoglobulin A abnormality: absence of light-heavy-chain assembly. Study of immunoglobulin synthesis in tonsillar cells. *J. Clin. Invest.*, **50**: 2526 (1971).

Naiman, J. L., Oski, F. A., Allen, F. H. and Diamond, L. K., Hereditary eosinophilia. *Am. J. Hum. Genet.*, **16**: 195 (1964).

Roberts, D. F. and Bradley, W. G., Immunoglobulin levels in dystrophia myotonica. *J. Med. Genet.*, **14**: 16 (1977).

Schimke, R. N., Horton, W. A. and King, C. R., Chondroitin-6-sulphaturia, defective cellular immunity, and nephrotic syndrome. *Lancet*, ii: 1088 (1971).

Soter, N. A., Wasserman, S. I. and Austen, K. F., Cold urticaria: release into the circulation of histamine and eosinophil chemotactic factor of anaphylaxis during cold challenge. *N. Engl. J. Med.*, **294**: 687 (1976).

Teisberg, P., Grottum, K. A., Myhre, E. and Flatmark, A., *In vivo* activation of complement in hereditary nephropathy. *Lancet*, ii: 356 (1973).

Appendix 1. Evaluation of the child with suspected immunological defects

Table A.1 lists some clinical problems in which the possibility of an underlying immunological defect should be suspected. Although they are categorized according to the system that is most involved, such a classification is frequently difficult in clinical practice. However, the study of the patient should be carried out progressively and according to the clinical picture, although in many cases this leads

Table A.1. Symptoms suggesting possible immunodeficiency.

1. B-cell defects
   (*a*) Recurrent pneumonia, meningitis or bacterial sepsis
   (*b*) Lymph-node hyperplasia
2. T-cell defects
   (*a*) Systemic disease following vaccination
   (*b*) Serious complications after a benign viral infection
   (*c*) Chronic oral candidiasis
   (*d*) Hypocalcaemia in the newborn period
3. Suggesting a combined T–B defect
   (*a*) Any combined symptomatology of T- and B-cell defects
   (*b*) Thrombocytopenia, eczema, ear infection (Wiskott-Aldrich)
   (*c*) Clinical manifestations of ataxia telangiectasia
   (*d*) Bone defects of the ADA deficiency
4. Suggesting complement defects
   (*a*) Recurrent pyogenic infectious (C3)
   (*b*) Seborrheic dermatitis (Leiner syndrome)
5. Suggesting phagocytic defects
   (*a*) Unexplained neutropenia
   (*b*) Pulmonary cyst; peculiar facies (Lichtenstein syndrome)
   (*c*) Chronic osteomyelitis
   (*d*) Suppurative lymphadenitis
6. Other
   (*a*) Ulcerative colitis in children
   (*b*) Pneumonia due to *N. carinii*
   (*c*) Intractable diarrhoea
   (*d*) Intractable eczema
   (*e*) Unexplained haematological disorder

to evaluation of the whole of the immune system. Besides the symptoms, other factors such as sex, family history, the site or sites of infection, and the organisms responsible need to be taken into account.

Evaluation of the humoral arm (B cells)

1. The measurement of immunoglobulin levels is obviously the simplest way of evaluating B cells. In general, any value less than 10% of the normal mean is considered as indicating a deficiency. It is of the utmost importance, therefore, to establish normal patterns for age for the population. Since there may be cases where the immunoglobulins are at normal levels but are not functional, one should consider the possibility of carrying out immunoelectrophoresis.

2. In doubtful cases, and particularly in the newborn and the nursing infant, functionality analysis can be carried out. The levels of isohaemagglutinins give an idea (except in children of type AB), although not a very precise one. More precise are the levels of antibodies after a vaccination, but it must be stressed that a suspicion of immune deficiency is an absolute contra-indication against vaccination of a child until it has been established whether deficiency exists and, if so, of what type.

The B-lymphocyte count may distinguish between the cases of cellular arrest and those due to a failure in the production or secretion of immunoglobulins.

Evaluation of the cellular arm

1. The lymphocyte count is usually the first indication of a defect at this level. Frequently lymphopenia accompanies the development of the immune deficiency but a normal count does not eliminate it.

2. The complete absence of thymus on thoracic X-rays indicates an immune deficiency at the T level. Its presence does not eliminate it.

3. Although a positive delayed cutaneous reaction indicates that the function of the macrophages and T cells is intact, a negative reaction may be due to various factors (i.e., no previous exposure to that antigen, deficiency at the level of the macrophage, a defect of T cells). The absence of previous exposure to the antigen can be excluded by repeating the test two weeks later.

4. The number of T cells as assessed by the total E rosettes is diminished in approximately half of the patients with cellular deficiencies. Examination of the subpopulations of T lymphocytes is sometimes useful.

5. Studies of T-cell function are more sophisticated, but also more precise. The proliferative response of the lymphocytes *in vitro* to phytohaemagglutinin and concanavalin-A is usually depressed in the cellular immunodeficiencies. One-way mixed-lymphocyte cultures are also usually hyporeactive in this type of immune deficiency.

6. Biopsy of the lymphatic nodes frequently shows cellular impoverishment in the T-dependent areas. In the same way, thymus biopsy may help to establish the diagnosis in these children.

Evaluation of the complement system

1. The complement system may be evaluated in various different ways. CH_{50} represents the sum of all the components of the system, but is not very sensitive to individual variations in any one of them.

2. If specific antibodies are available, it is possible to measure the levels of each of the components, but this does not show their functionality. Haemolytic tests are in this case more useful, but also technically more complicated. The activation of the complement system can be studied by two dimensional electrophoresis in which the conversion products of the components can be recognized.

3. Where there is deficiency of one or more of the isolated components, a family study should be made of the phenotypes and levels.

Appendix 2. Short notes on techniques in immunogenetics

This appendix does not pretend to be a laboratory manual, nor is it detailed enough to enable one to set up a particular technique. It is only intended to give an idea of the methods mentioned in the text and is an outline of some of the techniques that are available for assessing a patient with an immunological problem.

Radial immunodiffusion

This technique is based on the principle that a protein antigen diffuses radially from its point of application in a gel which contains antibodies to it and that a circular precipitate is formed at the point of equivalence. If the concentration of the antibody and the thickness of the gel are constant, the area covered by the precipitate is proportional to the concentration of the antigen. For the sake of convenience, the square of the diameter is used as the measure of this area. A graph of the concentration of the antigen against the square of the diameter is a straight line whose equation is $D^2 = K(CAG) + SO$, where D^2 is the square of the diameter, CAG the concentration of the antigen, and SO the point of intersection of the line with the Y co-ordinate.

All these calculations are not necessary if one uses commercially available plates for which there are also available control sera and standards. This technique is commonly used for measurement of the levels of immunoglobulins G, A and M and some of the components of complement.

Radioimmunoassay

Radioimmunoassay is a sensitive technique, but it requires experience and practice. Basically it is a competitive analysis, in which the protein that is going to be measured competes for a combination site with a known quantity of the same protein labelled with a radioisotope. After this competition for the antigen/antibody union, the free marked molecules are eliminated by centrifugation and the total

198

radiation of the precipitate is compared against the series of standards. In this way it is possible to calculate the amount of the marked protein which is joined to the antibody, and so to obtain indirectly a value corresponding to the amount of this protein in the sample analysed. This is the technique of choice for the measurement of proteins such as IgE and AFP which are normally found in very low concentrations.

Electrophoresis

Electrophoresis allows the identification of protein heterogeneity. There are various forms of electrophoresis with precise applications.

Zone Electrophoresis is the simplest form of electrophoresis, in which the proteins are separated only on the basis of their electric charge. Any support medium may be used such as agar, agarose, paper, cellulose acetate, etc., according to the proteins or group of proteins which it is required to separate. If agar or agarose are used as a support these should be prepared with a buffer that is either the same as that used for the bridge buffer (continuous electrophoresis) or different (discontinuous electrophoresis). Type of buffer, support medium, bridge material and duration of electrophoresis depend upon the type of protein to be analysed: for instance, for components of complement, agarose is usually used with a barbital buffer and continuous electrophoresis, while for adenosine deaminase and other enzymes starch is usually preferable.

Immunoelectrophoresis increases the analytical possibilities of zone electrophoresis. Initial separation of the proteins is carried out by the usual techniques of zone electrophoresis, and when this is completed a channel is made in the gel parallel to the direction of separation, and filled with antiserum for the proteins which are being investigated. There follows a reaction between the antigens present, separated in the zone electrophoresis, and the antibodies present in the antiserum, leading to precipitation in the zones of equivalence.

Radioimmuno-electrophoresis is a more sophisticated technique which combines electrophoresis with autoradiography. There are initial procedures *in vitro* before electrophoresis, for example, the addition of labelled amino acids to cultured cells. The cultured cells incorporate these amino acids in the synthesis of the protein, and the supernatant of these cultures is then submitted to normal electrophoresis followed by autoradiography.

Electro-immunodiffusion has two main forms: the double, or contrast, immunoelectrophoresis, and the simple, or rocket-electrophoresis of Laurel. Both are quite sensitive, but the simple has the advantage of being easier to quantify.

Evaluation of the complement system

There are many methods for the evaluation of the complement system. By means of radial immunodiffusion it is possible to measure the levels of almost all components, but not their functionality. This is why it is necessary to supplement these studies with others to show the activity of the total complement and each of its components.

CH_{50} **or haemolytic analysis** is a good method for studying the activity of the complement system, but has the disadvantage of not being very sensitive to individual variations in one or several of the components of the system. CH_{50} is an arbitrary measure that is defined as the quantity of complement necessary to lyse 50% of the erythrocytes sensitized with antibodies.

Functional assays of the components of complement are based on a similar scheme to that of CH_{50}, but utilizing serum that is deficient in the component that it is required to measure. Serum of the patient is added to the sensitized red cells, followed by serum deficient in the component under study. If that component is functional in the patient's serum there will be haemolysis.

Studies in cellular immunity *in vitro*

There are two classic analyses to measure cellular immunity *in vitro*. The first, migration inhibition, measures the production of the factor inhibiting migration; the second, lymphocyte transformation, measures the response of the lymphocytes to stimulation by specific and non-specific antigens.

The migration-inhibition test measures the production of the inhibitor factor of migration by its effects on a target-cell population which may be macrophages or monocytes. This technique is based on the observation that the cells of the peritoneal exudate of a sensitized animal (which are usually 70% macrophages and 20% lymphocytes) when placed in a capillary tube tend to move upwards in the tube. This migratory tendency can be inhibited by adding the sensitizing antigen to the culture medium in which the macrophages were incubated, since this leads to the production of the migration-inhibiting factor. There are various ways of carrying out this test, using cells of the guinea-pig, human leukocytes, or a combination of both.

Transformation or activation of lymphocytes measures the functional capacity of the lymphocyte to proliferate after antigenic stimulation. The technique is basically as follows: lymphocytes are separated from peripheral blood by density-gradient centrifugation in ficoll hypaque and triplicate cultures are established with an adequate cell concentration (1×10^6 lymphocytes per ml). The mitogens or antigens are added to this culture and incubated for 72 hours in an atmosphere containing 5% CO_2, then tritiated thymidine is added to the cultures, which will be incorporated by the DNA recently synthesized; this rate of DNA synthesis is then measured in a scintillation counter. There are obviously a variety of technical problems in this method.

Mixed-lymphocyte culture is one of the several techniques used to measure the activation of the lymphocyte, but it can also be used for examining the immune competence of the T cells, as well as the analysis of the histocompatibility antigens related to the *D* locus. In mixed-lymphocyte culture, the stimulating factor is provided by the histocompatibility antigens on the surface of other lymphocytes. This test may be carried out with either one-way or two-way stimulation. In one-way culture, one of the cell populations is treated by radiation or mitomycin-C to inhibit the synthesis of DNA, while retaining the capacity for the antigenic stimulation. In this case, one measures only the synthesizing capacity of the DNA in the other cell population. In two-way mixed-lymphocyte culture, both cell populations are equally viable and both of them therefore respond in the synthesis of DNA.

HLA typing: microlymphocytotoxicity techniques

The technique of Kisssmeyer-Nielsen and Kjerbye is commonly the routine technique for typing *HLA-A, -B* and *-C*, and has recently come into use for typing the *DR* locus.

This procedure is carried out in microplates in which are placed 1 ml of antiserum and 1 ml of the lymphocyte suspension (approximately 1×10^6 cells per ml in a mixture of 1 : 1 normal human serum and complement). After careful mixture, incubation is carried out for 30 minutes at $37\,^\circ$C, and then 0.5 μl of 1% trypan blue is added, and again incubated for 30 minutes at room temperature. Reading is carried out under normal lighting with an inverted microscope. Dead cells (those which have taken up the blue stain) are counted and are scored as follows (Figure A.8):

15–25% dead cells	+
26–55% dead cells	+ +
56–80% dead cells	+ + +
81–100% dead cells	+ + + +

The modified technique of the National Institutes of Health is the best technique for typing *DR*. In general, the procedure is very similar to the previous one. In the wells of the microplates are placed 0.5 μl of antiserum and 0.5 μl of the cell suspension in culture medium (concentration 2×10^2 per ml), followed by incubation for 30 minutes at $20\,^\circ$C. Then 2.5 μl of rabbit complement are added and further incubation is carried out at $20\,^\circ$C for 60 minutes. Then trypan blue is added (0.5 μl of 1.8% trypan blue) and reading is done after further incubation at $20\,^\circ$C for 30–45 minutes.

The mixed-lymphocyte reaction, already described for measuring the activation of the lymphocyte, is the *in vitro* technique which allows the detection of *D* locus differences but with a minor variation. The stimulating cells are those of an individual who, by family study, has been shown to be a homozygote for a gene at the *D* locus. Any cell with the same specificity at the *D* locus will not incorporate tritiated thymidine when brought into contact with the homozygous typing cells.

Evaluation of phagocytic function

There are various tests for the measurement of phagocytic function.

Separation of the polymorphonuclear neutrophils is usually done from heparinized venous blood. By sedimentation, the red cells are separated, and the supernatant which is rich in leukocytes is transferred to a conical plastic tube, where the preparation can be freed of contamination with (*a*) red cells by hypotonic lysis, (*b*) platelets by differential centrifugation, (*c*) lymphocytes and mononucleocytes by centrifugation through the density gradients in ficoll hypaque.

The cellular adherence of the polymorphonuclear cells can easily be measured by passing the suspension of cells through a microcolumn of glass fibre. In this test, the percentage of neutrophils which adhere to the nylon column is measured by counting the cells before and after the passage through the column.

Chemotaxis is assessed by measuring the ability of the polymorphonuclear cells to move towards a chemotactic stimulus. One of the methods most frequently used is that of the Boyden chamber. This chamber consists of a lower receptacle full of chemotactic agent, above which a micropore filter is placed with a leukocyte suspension. To establish a chemotactic gradient, a chamber with a buffer is placed on top. Frequently it requires incubation for three hours, then the cells are stained, and the number of cells which have migrated through the filter established.

Phagocytic ingestion is measured by the percentage of ingestion of red O oil by the polymorphonuclear neutrophils. Briefly, the phagocytic cells are placed in contact with lipopolysaccharides of *Escherichia coli*, covered with paraffin and stained with red O oil, then after incubation, during which the phagocytes have absorbed part of these lipopolysaccharides, the red O oil is extracted from the cells and is measured by spectrophotometry.

Oxidase activation is measured in many ways which reflect reactivation of oxidase by the neutrophil during phagocytosis. The test of nitro-blue tetrazolium (NTB) is based on the fact that during phagocytosis the neutrophil reduces the nitro-blue tetrazolium to formazan due to the presence of activated oxygen in the cell. In short, the test is done by adding nitro-blue tetrazolium which is yellow to a phagocyte suspension. This is incubated for 15 minutes and then it is possible to observe the red colour of the formazan in the phagocytic vesicles. The patients with problems at this level of phagocytosis (e.g., chronic granulomatous disease) do not reduce the NTB after 15 minutes of incubation.

Bacteriocidal analysis *in vitro* is a test that is essential in any patient in whom a defect of microbicidal activity is suspected. In peroxidative killing generally, equal amounts of neutrophils and bacteria are incubated with fresh serum at 10% as a source of opsonins. Incubation is carried out at 37°C for 120 minutes. Then aliquots from the tubes of the patient and the control are taken at intervals of 30 minutes, diluted in sterile tubes, and mixed with Agar in a petri dish. These dishes are incubated for 12 hours, after which the bacterial colonies are counted.

Glossary

Activated lymphocyte	A lymphocyte stimulated by an antigen or mitogen.
Adenosinedeaminase (ADA)	Enzyme which catalyses the conversion of adenosine to inosine.
Agglutination	Formation of aggregations, usually of red cells.
Allele	One of the two genes at a given locus which control a particular character.
Alloantigen	Surface antigens which differ from one individual to another in the same species.
Allogenic	Relationship which exists between two members of the same species, possibly genetically different.
Allotransplant	Transplant between two members of the same species, possibly genetically different.
Allotype	The antigenic differences of genetically determined proteins which show variations between members of the same species.
Alphafoetoprotein (AFP)	Protein or antigen to which has been assigned a possible immunosuppressive effect *in vitro*, useful in the prenatal diagnosis of neural-tube defects.
Alternate pathway	Pathway of activation of complement from C3 without involving specific antibodies.
Am marker	Allotypic determinants of the H chain of human IgA.
Amorph	A gene which does not apparently produce an antigenic determinant.
Antibody	A generic term for the immunoglobulin produced as the result of the presence of an antigen, and which has the capacity to combine with it.
Antibody-dependent cell cytotoxicity	A cell-mediated form of cytotoxicity in which an effector cell destroys a white cell covered with antibodies.

Antigen	Substance capable of provoking an immune response.
Antigenic determinant	The area of an antigen against which an immune response is mounted (= epitope).
Anti-lymphocytic serum	One possessing antibodies against lymphocytes.
Antiserum	A suspension of antibodies.
Autoantibodies	Antibodies against the carrier's own antigens.
Autoimmunity	Immunity against one's own antigens.
Autosomal dominant	An allele which is shown phenotypically in the heterozygotes.
Autosomal recessive	Mode of inheritance in which an allele is only expressed phenotypically in the homozygote.
Autosome	A chromosome not involved in sex differentiation.
Balanced polymorphism	Polymorphism which is stabilized usually as a result of selective advantage of the heterozygote.
Beta-2 microglobulin	Light chain associated with some of the products of the major histocompatibility system.
Bimodal distribution	A distribution of events characterized by two peaks.
B lymphocyte	Cells which take their origin from the bursar or its equivalent. They are the precursors of the plasmocytes.
Bonferroni inequality	A situation in which simultaneous statistical testing of many associations causes a number of them to reach a conventionally significant level by pure chance.
Camptodactyly	Malformation of the hand characterized by a contraction deformity of the proximal interphalangeal articulations of the digits.
Cell hybridization	Crossing of cells of different origins.
Centimorgan (cM)	Unit of distance between two genes: 1cM = 1% probability of recombination.
Centromere	Portion of the chromosome by which it is attached to the spindle in cell division.
Chemotaxis	Chemical process which attracts phagocytes to the site of infection.
Chimerism	Presence of an individual with cell lines of different genotype.
Chromosomal aberration	A chromosomal defect visible under the light microscope.
Chromosomal inversion	A chromosomal aberration produced when a chromosome breaks at two places and the part between the breaks is reinserted after rotation.

Classes of immunoglobulins	Subdivision of the molecules of immunoglobulins dependent on the constitution of the heavy chain.
Classic pathway	Pathway of activation of complement from C1.
Clone	Group of cells deriving from a single cell.
Co-dominant	Form of heredity in which the two alleles are both expressed in the heterozygote.
Complement	System of proteins acting in a cascade with the function of destroying antigens covered with antibodies.
Concanavalin A	Lectin which preferentially stimulates T lymphocytes.
Congenic	Line of mice genetically identical to each other except at a histocompatibility locus.
Correlation coefficient	Coefficient which measures the degree of variation of a series of points from a straight line in a Cartesian diagram.
C region	The portion of the carboxyl terminal of the H or L chain which shows variations in its amino acid sequence.
Crossing over	Process of exchange of genetic information between two homologous chromosomes.
Cryoglobulin	Protein that can be precipitated by freezing.
Cytotoxic reaction	Cellular action of complement or other agents which lead to cell death.
Degranulation	Process in which the cytoplasmic granules of phagocytes combine with the phagosome and are destroyed.
Delayed cutaneous hypersensitivity	Cell-mediated immune reaction when an antigen is introduced subcutaneously.
Deletion	Absence of segment of a chromosome.
Disulphide bonds	Chemical bonds between amino acids which contain the sulphydril group.
Domains	Segments of the immunoglobulin chains which are stabilized by disulphide bonds.
Down's syndrome	Trisomy 21 or mongolism.
Effector cells	T cells capable of producing cytotoxic, suppressor or helper functions.
Epistasis	Non-additive interaction between two or more loci.
E rosettes	Aggregation of sheep erythrocytes with T lymphocytes.
Exon	Segment of a gene which is expressed in messenger RNA and is a coding region.
Fab fragment	Fragment of immunoglobulin produced by

	papain digestion which has the capacity of antigen combination.
Familial aggregation	The occurrence in the same family of several cases of a disorder which are not necessarily inherited as Mendelian characters.
Fc fragment	Fragment of the immunoglobulin produced by digestion with papain which contains the carboxyl terminal part of the two heavy chains.
Fc receptor	Receptor for the Fc fragment of the immunoglobulin present on the surface of various cell types.
Gamma globulin	Serum protein of the electrophoretic gamma fraction, among which occur the immunoglobulins.
Gene	DNA segment with a detectable function.
Gene frequency	The proportion in which an allele is found in the gene pool of a given population.
Genotype	The genetic consitution of an individual.
Genetic heterogeneity	Situation where what is apparently a single clinical entity is found to consist of two or more genotypically distinct.
Genetic marker	Genetic characteristic used in the chromosomal assignation of genes or in the definition of genetic heterogeneity.
Germ cells	Gametes or their precursors.
Germ line	The cell line which produces gametes.
Gm marker	Allotypic determinant of the heavy chain of human IgG.
Graft-versus-host disease	Clinical manifestation of the reaction mounted by immunocompetent cells of the host against the cells of the transplant.
H-2	The major histocompatibility system of the mouse.
Haplotype	Combination of genetic determinants localized on the same chromosome and closely linked.
Hardy-Weinberg law	Rule predicting the genotype frequencies from the gene frequencies in a population.
Heavy chain (H)	Polypeptide chain which determines the class of immunoglobulin.
Helper T cells	Subpopulation of T cells which co-operate with the B cells in the formation of antibodies.
Heritability	The fraction of the total variance due to genes as distinct from that due to environmental factors.
Heterologous	Relation which usually denotes antigenic differences between two species.

Heterozygote	A carrier of different alleles at a locus.
HLA	Abbreviation of Human Leucocyte Antigen, the human major histocompatibility system.
Homozygote	One in whom both alleles at a locus are the same.
Humoral immunity	Immunity mediated by antibodies.
Hypervariable regions	Segments of pronounced variation in the V region of heavy and light chains, responsible for the specificity of the molecule.
Hypogammaglobulinaemia	Deficiency of all the classes of serum immunoglobulins.
Idiotype	An antigenic determinant characteristic of the type of antibody and of a myeloma protein.
IgT	Immunoglobulin present theoretically on the surface of T cells.
Immunization	Process which causes an individual to produce antibodies.
Immunoglobulin subclasses	Subdivision of the classes of immunoglobulin based on structural or antigenic differences of the H chain.
Incompatibility	The presence in the foetus, transplant or insert, of an antigenic substance which provokes an immune response in the mother or recipient.
Interferon	Heterogeneous group of proteins produced by cells infected by a virus.
Intron	Segment of the gene which is not expressed in messenger RNA and which has no coding function.
In vitro	Experiments carried out with cultured cells in the laboratory.
In vivo	Experiments and observations carried out in the living organism.
Ir gene	Gene which controls the immune response to a specific antigen.
Iso-	(Isologous, isogenic, etc.) Denotes genetic identity. Syngenic is synonymous with isogenic.
Isoantibodies	Antibodies which react with an antigen present in another member of the same species.
Isochromosome	Chromosome with morphologically identical arms.
Isohaemagglutinins	Antibodies against the red cells of individuals of the same species.
Karyotype	The chromosomal array.
Killer cells	Cells with antibody-dependent cellular cytotoxicity.

Light chain (L) Polypeptide chain associated with the heavy chain of the immunoglobulins.

Linkage The presence of two or more genes close together on the same chromosome, manifested by the tendency for them to be transmitted together.

Linkage disequilibrium Situation in which two or more genes closely linked occur together in the same haplotype at greater frequencies than expected from the frequency of each individually.

Locus Position of a gene on a chromosome.

Lod score Acronym for logarithm of the odds ratio. Statistical method which allows linkage studies in families.

Major histocompatibility system Group of linked genes which determine surface antigens and other protein fractions with histocompatibility functions.

Mitogen Substance which activates cell division.

Mixed lymphocyte culture *In vitro* technique in which the mixture of lymphocytes from two individuals stimulates their proliferation.

Mosaic Presence in an individual of two or more cell lines of different genotype, produced by mutation or a chromosomal aberration.

Opsonification Process of covering an antigen with antibodies.

Phagocyte Cell capable of ingesting phagosomes.

Phenotype External manifestation of the genotype.

Phytohaemagglutinin Mitogen which principally stimulates proliferation of T lymphocytes.

Pokeweed Mitogen of vegetable origin which stimulates T and B lymphocytes to proliferate.

Polygenic inheritance Influenced by the cumulative effect of many genes.

Polymorphism Existence of two or more alleles at a given locus in a population, so that the least common is present at a frequency of more than 1%.

Polyploid duplication Mechanism by which a defect in meiosis results in the duplication of one or more chromosomes.

Proband or propositus (Feminine proposita, plural propositi or propositae.) Patient through whom a family is ascertained.

Quantitative character Character showing continuous variation.

Recombinant The individual in whom it is possible to detect crossing over, or the characteristic which has recombined.

Recombination	The result of crossing over.
Recombination frequency	Average frequency of crossing over between two loci.
Regulator gene	Gene which controls the function of the operon and thereby structural genes whose action depends upon the operator gene.
Relative risk	Terms in which it is usual to express the association between a genetic marker and a disorder.
Sex linked	Determined by genes located on the sex chromosome.
Site of antigenic combination	Part of the immunoglobulin responsible for its union with the antigen.
Structural gene	Gene responsible for the production of a specific chemical structure.
Svedberg unit	Measure of the sedimentation velocity of a molecule or particle in a gravitational field.
Tandem duplication	Mechanism by which crossing over in meiosis results in the elongation of a DNA segment and duplication of one or several genes.
T-dependent antigen	Antigen which necessitates the collaboration of T with B cells in order to produce antibodies.
Tetraploidy	Condition in which there is four times the haploid number of chromosomes.
Translocation	Chromosomal aberration in which all of a chromosome or part of it is joined to another.
Xenogenic	Between members of different species.

Index